O C L
OXFORD CARDIOLOGY LIBRARY

Lipid Disorders

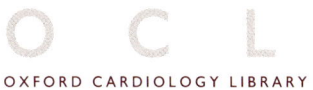

OXFORD CARDIOLOGY LIBRARY

Lipid Disorders

Paul Nicholls

Consultant Physician and Honorary
Professor of Medicine,
Royal Victoria Hospital, Belfast

Ian Young

Professor of Medicine and Consultant
Clinical Biochemist,
Queen's University of Belfast and
Royal Victoria Hospital, Belfast

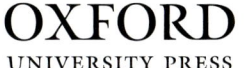

OXFORD
UNIVERSITY PRESS

OXFORD
UNIVERSITY PRESS

Great Clarendon Street, Oxford OX2 6DP

Oxford University Press is a department of the University of Oxford.
It furthers the University's objective of excellence in research, scholarship,
and education by publishing worldwide in

Oxford New York

Auckland Cape Town Dar es Salaam Hong Kong Karachi
Kuala Lumpur Madrid Melbourne Mexico City Nairobi
New Delhi Shanghai Taipei Toronto

With offices in

Argentina Austria Brazil Chile Czech Republic France Greece
Guatemala Hungary Italy Japan Poland Portugal Singapore
South Korea Switzerland Thailand Turkey Ukraine Vietnam

Oxford is a registered trade mark of Oxford University Press
in the UK and in certain other countries

Published in the United States
by Oxford University Press Inc., New York

British Library Cataloguing in Publication Data

Data available

Library of Congress Cataloging in Publication Data

Data available

Typeset by Newgen Imaging Systems (P) Ltd., Chennai, India
Printed in Great Britain
on acid-free paper by
Ashford Colour Press Ltd., Gosport, Hants

ISBN 978-0-19-956965-6

10 9 8 7 6 5 4 3 2 1

Contents

We are grateful to the staff of the Lipid Clinic, to Dr Colin Graham and the staff of the Regional Molecular Genetics Laboratory, and to the patients themselves for making the clinic a stimulating environment in which to work.

Preface

The Lipid Clinic at the Royal Victoria Hospital was founded in 1972 by Dr Richard Womersley. At that time, lipidology was a Cinderella speciality, and events of the 1980s did not improve this perception. With the advent of effective treatment in the form of statins, interest was renewed and has continued to grow. The management of lipid disorders now interfaces with many specialities, including primary care, and within the hospital, Cardiology, Vascular Medicine, Neurology, Diabetes, and Clinical Chemistry. The present book is intended to improve understanding of the current views on this topic, in a useful pocket format. It is intended to complement, not to replace, the standard textbooks, which will continue to provide a valuable reference source. We hope it will prove to be helpful to a wide audience of non-specialists.

Paul Nicholls
Ian Young

Abbreviations

ABCA-1	adenosine triphosphate-binding cassette protein A1
ACAT	acyl CoA cholesteryl acyl transferase
ACS	acute coronary syndromes
AIDS	acquired immunodeficiency syndrome
ALT	alanine aminotransferase
AST	aspartate aminotransferase
CETP	cholesteryl ester transfer protein
CHD	coronary heart disease
CoQ10	ubiquinone coenzyme Q10
CK	creatine kinase
tCK	total creatine kinase
CKD	chronic kidney disease
CVD	cardiovascular disease
ESC	European Society for Cardiology
ESRD	end-stage renal disease
FCH	familial combined hyperlipidaemia
FDA	Food and Drug Administration
FDB	familial dysbetalipoproteinaemia
FH	familial hypercholesterolaemia
γGT	gamma-glutamyl transpeptidase
HDL	high-density lipoprotein
HDL-C	high-density lipoprotein cholesterol
HeFH	heterozygous familial hypercholesterolaemia
HIV	human immunodeficiency virus
HoFH	homozygous familial hypercholesterolaemia
HMG-CoA	β-hydroxy-β-methylglutaryl-coenzyme A
IDL	intermediate density lipoprotein
IVUS	intravascular ultrasound
JBS	Joint British Societies
LCAT	lecithin cholesterol acyltransferase
LDL	low-density lipoprotein
LDL-C	low-density lipoprotein cholesterol

Lp(a)	lipoprotein (a)
Lp-PLA$_2$	lipoprotein-associated phospholipase
MCV	mean corpuscular volume
MI	myocardial infarction
NAFLD	non-alcoholic fatty liver disease
NASH	non-alcoholic steatohepatitis
NICE	National Institute for Health and Clinical Excellence
NSTEMI	non-ST elevation MI
TC	total cholesterol
TG	triglyceride
TRL	TG-rich lipoproteins
TX	tendon xanthomata
VLDL	very low density lipoprotein

Chapter 1

History of lipids

Key points
- The association of cholesterol and atheroma has been known for many years.
- Only recently has effective treatment become available.
- Such treatment is now in widespread use.

The concept that fat is present in the blood has been recognized for over 200 yrs, since it was first noted that blood plasma turned milky after food (see Table 1.1). Cholesterol became one of the first organic molecules to be identified, and the association of cholesterol, atheroma, and skin deposits was described in the 19th century. In the early 20th century, cholesterol was one of the few molecules that could be measured in blood, and was used as a biomarker for hypothyroidism long before thyroid hormones could be measured.

The association of high cholesterol levels and increased risk of coronary heart disease (CHD) was recognized from epidemiological studies in the 1950s, but at that time treatment options were limited to resins or nicotinic acid, and so the hypothesis that cholesterol reduction would also reduce CHD could not be tested.

The first drug specifically designed to reduce lipids was clofibrate, introduced in 1962 by ICI Pharmaceuticals (now Astra Zeneca).

Table 1.1 Landmarks in the history of lipid disorders

- von Haller (1755)—'atheroma' in arteries
- Hewson (1771)—alimentary lipaemia in dogs
- Chevreul (1816)—identification of the cholesterol molecule
- Vogel (1845)—cholesterol present in atheroma
- Fagge (1873)—xanthomata and atheroma
- Anitschow (1913)—lipids and atheroma
- de Langen (1916)—cholesterol and diet
- Burns (1920)—clinical features of HeFH
- Havel (1955)—ultracentrifugation of lipids
- Keys (1961)—epidemiology of cholesterol
- ICI Pharmaceuticals (1962)—clofibrate
- WHO trial (1978)
- Nobel Prize to Goldstein and Brown (1985)
- 4S study (1994)

In order to test the hypothesis that cholesterol reduction would reduce the incidence of CHD, the first major multicentre international trial was set up under the direction of the World Health Organisation (WHO). The report of this trial in 1978 (see Chapter 12) indicated that clofibrate produced a significant reduction in coronary events, but at the expense of an increase in all-cause mortality. This caused widespread scepticism that cholesterol reduction would be of any benefit, although it is now thought that the WHO trial suffered from problems of data inclusion and analysis. Nevertheless the negative view prevailed, despite other major trials such as the Lipid Research Clinic and the Coronary Drug Project studies in the USA, and the Helsinki Heart Study from Europe. A summary of these and other studies may also be found in Chapter 12.

Two other areas for concern were prevalent at this time. First was an apparent increase in cancer mortality at low levels of cholesterol, which led to doubts about reducing cholesterol levels. A 'J'- or 'U'-shaped curve of cholesterol vs mortality had been noted in at least two major studies (LRC-CPPT, 1984; Martin et al., 1986). The apparent increase in mortality at low levels of cholesterol is almost certainly due to the minority in the population with asymptomatic malignant diseases or infections (Rose and Shipley, 1980; Sherwin et al., 1987). Long-term safety data on statins have not shown any increased cancer risk over a 20-year period (Chapter 9). Second, both the LRC-CPPT of 1984 and the Helsinki Heart Study (Frick et al., 1987) suggested that there could be an increase in suicide or violent deaths in the group on active treatment. In fact, the numbers were small, and did not reach statistical significance (11 vs 4 and 9 vs 5, respectively). A description of the individual deaths makes an association with lipid-lowering treatment implausible (Wysowski and Gross, 1990), and again this relationship has not been confirmed in later studies.

In 1985, the Nobel Prize for Medicine was awarded to Joseph Goldsmith and Michael Brown from Dallas for their discovery of the role of 3-hydroxymethyl-3-glutaryl coenzyme A (HMG-CoA) reductase in the synthetic pathway of cholesterol in the liver (Goldstein and Brown, 1977), and the role of low-density lipoprotein (LDL) receptors in the clearance of cholesterol from the blood (Goldstein and Brown, 1975). These fundamental discoveries led to the development of inhibitors of HMG-CoA reductase (statins) (Endo et al., 1976).

These drugs were able to reduce circulating cholesterol levels by 25% or more and therefore enabled the cholesterol hypothesis to be retested. The publication of the Scandinavian Simvastatin Survival Study (4S) in 1994 was a landmark as it established beyond dispute that cholesterol reduction in men with CHD (secondary prevention) reduced both morbidity and mortality. Other major studies such as WOSCOPS (primary prevention) and CARE followed soon after (see Chapter 12) and together provide the scientific background to the guidelines on cholesterol treatment from the Joint British Societies (JBS), the National Institute for Health and Clinical Excellence (NICE), and others (see Chapters 6 and 9).

References

Endo A, Kuroda M, and Tsujitsa Y (1976). ML-236A, ML-236B, and ML-236C, new inhibitors of cholesterogenesis produced by *Penicillium citrinum*. *J. Antibiot. (Tokyo)*, **29**, 1346–8.

Frick MH, Elo O, Haapa K et al. (1987). Helsinki Heart Study. *N. Engl. J. Med.*, **317**, 1237–45.

Goldstein JL and Brown MS (1975). Familial hypercholesterolemia: a genetic regulatory defect in cholesterol metabolism. *Am. J. Med.*, **58**, 147–50.

Goldstein JL and Brown MS (1977). The low-density lipoprotein pathway and its relation to atherosclerosis. *Ann. Rev. Biochem.*, **46**, 897–930.

Lipid Research Clinics Program Coronary Primary Prevention Trial. LRC Program (1984). *J. Am. Med. Assoc.*, **251**, 351–64.

Martin MJ, Hulley SB, Browner WS, Kuller LH, and Wentworth D (1986). Serum cholesterol, blood pressure and mortality: implications from a cohort of 361 662 men. *Lancet*, **ii**, 933–6.

Rose G and Shipley MJ (1980). Plasma lipids and mortality: a source of error. *Lancet*, **i**, 523–6.

Scandinavian Simvastatin Survival Study (1994). *Lancet*, **344**, 1383–9.

Sherwin RW, Wentworth DD, Cutler JA et al. (1987). Serum cholesterol levels and cancer mortality in 361 662 men screened for the Multiple Risk Factor Intervention Trial. *J. Am. Med. Assoc.*, **257**, 943–8.

Wysowski DK and Gross TP (1990). Deaths due to accidents and violence in two recent trials of cholesterol-lowering drugs. *Ann. Intern. Med.*, **150**, 2169–72.

Chapter 2

Epidemiology

Key points

- Total and low-density lipoprotein cholesterol (LDL-C) levels are inappropriately high in the developed world.
- Levels can be linked to the prevalence of coronary heart disease (CHD).
- Triglyceride (TG) levels are also associated with an increased risk of CHD, especially when coupled with low levels of high-density lipoprotein cholesterol (HDL-C).
- CHD event rates are declining in Western Europe, and increasing in Eastern Europe.

2.1 Introduction

Of the major lipid components, cholesterol is essential for many body functions (see Table 2.1) and TG is a valuable calorie-rich fuel. Both are present in all mammalian species, but total cholesterol (TC) levels rarely exceed 4 mmol (or LDL-C > 2 mmol/L) except in man (O'Keefe et al., 2004). The minimum amount biologically necessary in man is not known, but many populations in the Third World have circulating LDL-C levels of 2 mmol/L or less, levels which were probably present in our hunter–gatherer ancestors (O'Keefe et al., 2004; Kirby, 2008). The effects of LDL-C reduction on cardiovascular events in the major studies can be extrapolated backwards to indicate a similar ideal level (Figure 2.1) (Stamler et al., 2000; O'Keefe et al., 2004; LaRosa al., 2005). In theory, LDL-C levels of 0.8 mmol/L (primary prevention) or 1.5 mmol/L (secondary prevention) would be associated with a zero event rate.

Table 2.1 Cholesterol is necessary

- Membrane structure, especially brain
- Bile acid formation
- Lipoprotein formation
- Steroid hormones including cortisol, aldosterone, and sex hormones
- Vitamin D formation
- Regulatory actions

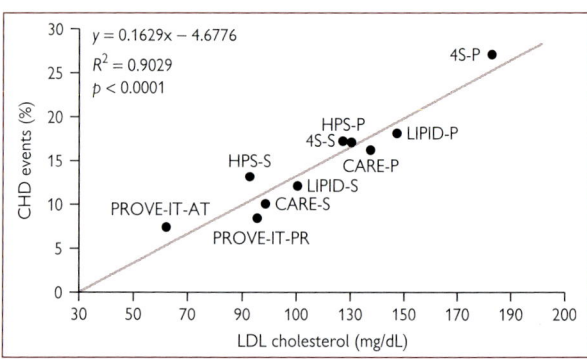

Figure 2.1 Effects of LDL-C reduction on CHD mortality, linear relationship of LDL-C reduction and CHD events.

In the Western world and other 'developed' countries, the circulating levels of TC are often much higher. In the UK, the mean level in men was 5.9 mmol/L 20 yrs ago (Mann *et al.*, 1988), and is probably much the same now. The 'normal' level of TC (i.e. the population mean ± 2 standard deviations) is therefore not the same as the 'ideal' or 'desirable' level, nor indeed the target level for treatment.

TC levels are low after trauma, operations, malignancy, and major illness such as acute myocardial infarction or stroke (catabolic phase). TC levels are not significantly affected by recent food intake and so samples do not have to be taken fasting, although fasting samples are required for the accurate measurement of LDL-C, HDL-C, and TG.

2.2 **Cholesterol in different countries**

The relationship between cholesterol levels and CHD mortality in different countries has been recognized for many years (Keys, 1975) and is backed up by large single population studies such as the Lipid Research Clinics Program (1979), Framingham (Dawber, 1980), and MrFIT (1982). In the Ni-Hon-San study (Kagan *et al.*, 1974), Japanese people who emigrated eastwards to Honolulu and then California increased their TC levels and their CHD mortality despite a decrease in blood pressure and smoking, indicating the importance of environmental effects, especially a change in diet.

Figure 2.1 is reproduced from O'Keefe, *et al.*, (2004). Optimal low-density lipoprotein is 50 to 70 mg/dl: Lower is better and physiologically normal. *J. Am. Coll. Cardiol.*, **43**: 2142–6, with permission from Elsevier, © 2004.

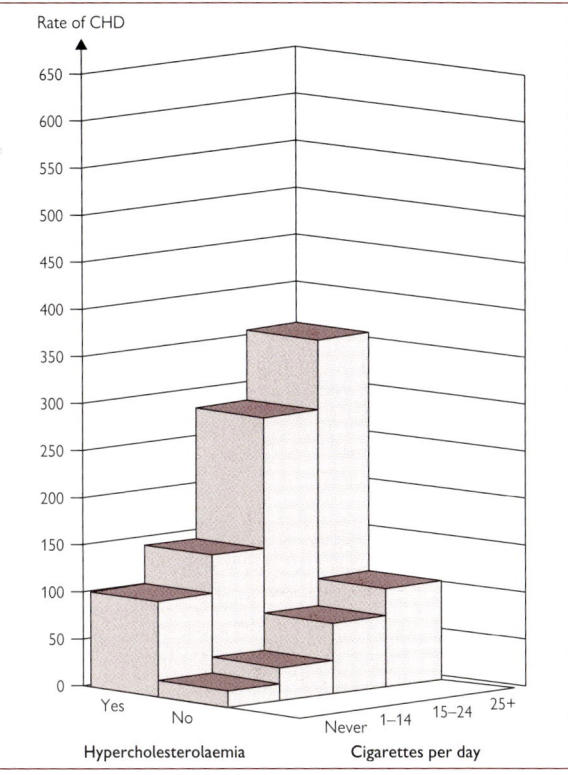

Figure 2.2 Smoking and hypercholesterolaemia. Study in >100,000 American nurses with raised (>6.2 mmol/L) or 'normal' cholesterol (<6.2 mmol/L): relationship of cardiovascular risk and number of cigarettes smoked daily.

2.3 **Interacting risk factors**

The dynamic interlink of the four key CHD risk factors (hyperlipidaemia, hypertension, diabetes, and cigarette smoking) means that any study involving just one of these has to be interpreted with caution (Willett et al., 1987) (see Figure 2.2). In addition, it is important to distinguish between primary prevention (no known vascular disease) and secondary prevention, which includes not only those with known vascular disease, but also those at high risk (diabetes, severe

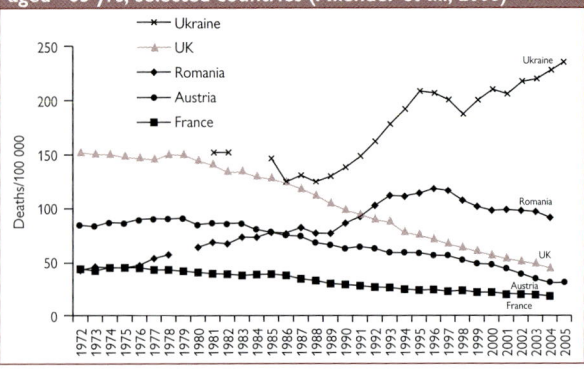

Figure 2.3 Deaths from CHD in Europe, 1972 to 2005. Males aged <65 yrs, selected countries (Allender et al., 2008)

hypertension, and inherited dyslipidaemias such as heterozygous familial hypercholesterolaemia (HeFH) and familial combined hyperlipidaemia (FCH)).

2.4 **Changing patterns of disease**

The prevalence of CHD is gradually declining in Western countries, and increasing in other areas, especially in Russia and Eastern European states (Allender et al., 2008). The age-standardized death rates from CHD in men aged 64 or less has fallen in the UK from 151 in 1972 to 44 in 2004 (see Figure 2.3). A similar reduction has been observed in women (36 to 11 over the same time period). The rate in men has risen in Russia from 169 in 1980 to 242 in 2005, so that it is now the leading country for CHD deaths. The lowest rate is in France (17 in 2004). Furthermore, the pattern of CHD in Europe is changing, with fewer myocardial infarcts and more acute coronary syndromes.

2.5 **TGs and CHD**

It is more difficult to establish a relationship between serum TGs and CHD. In part, this is due to wide fluctuations in TG concentrations throughout the day, the heterogeneity of TG-rich lipoproteins (TRL), and the inseparable correlations between TG and other CVD risk factors. Nevertheless, several studies have established a clear relationship of TGs to CHD, independent of HDL-C (Carlson et al., 1979; Castelli, 1986, Criqui et al., 1993; Hokanson and Austin, 1996).

It was estimated that raised TG levels were associated with a 13% increase in CVD risk in men and a 37% increase in women following adjustment for confounding factors. TGs were found to have a strong inverse correlation with HDL-C, although the association between TGs and CVD was independent of this relationship.

A more sophisticated approach to examining the physiological impact of TGs is to analyse the individual TRL, which is a broad term encompassing chylomicrons, very low density lipoprotein (VLDL), and their partially metabolized remnant lipoproteins, a heterogeneous population of particles with wide-ranging atherogenic potential. Accumulating evidence suggests that elevated plasma TGs, in the form of TRL, are independent cardiovascular risk factors with an atherogenic potential comparable to raised LDL.

2.6 HDL-C and CHD

In contrast to TC, LDL, and TGs, HDL-C concentration has an inverse association with CVD (Assmann et al., 1998; see Chapters 4 and 6). The anti-atherogenic properties of HDL-C have been accounted for by the involvement of HDL in reverse cholesterol transport. However, HDL has numerous functions independent from lipid metabolism which are protective against atherogenesis, including anti-inflammatory properties and an ability to protect LDL against oxidation (Ansell et al., 2004). In general, risk is greatest at HDL-C levels of less than 1.0 mmol/L in men and 1.2 mmol/L in women (UK HDL-C Consensus Group, 2004).

References

Allender S, Scarborough P, Peto V et al. (2008). European cardiovascular disease statistics. European Heart Network, Belgium.

Ansell BJ, Navab M, Watson KE, Fonarow GC, and Fogelman AM (2004). Anti-inflammatory properties of HDL. Rev. Endocr. Metab. Disord., 5, 351–8.

Assmann G, Cullen P, and Schulte H (1998). The Munster Heart Study (PROCAM). Results of follow-up at 8 years. Eur. Heart J., 19 (Suppl. A), A2–A11.

Carlson LA, Bottiger LE, and Ahfeldt PE (1979). Risk factors for myocardial infarction in the Stockholm Prospective Study. A 14-year follow-up focussing on the role of plasma triglycerides and cholesterol. Acta Med. Scand., 206, 351–60.

Castelli WP (1986). The triglyceride issue: a view from Framingham. Am. Heart J., 112, 432–7.

Criqui MH, Heiss G, Cohn R et al. (1993). Plasma triglyceride level and mortality from coronary heart disease. N. Eng. J. Med., 328: 1120–5

Dawber TR (1980). *The Framingham Study. The epidemiology of atherosclerotic disease.* Harvard University Press, Cambridge, MA.

Hokanson JE and Austin MA (1996). Plasma triglyceride level is a risk factor for cardiovascular disease independent of high-density lipoprotein cholesterol level: a meta-analysis of population-based prospective studies. *J. Cardiovasc. Risk*, **3**, 213–9.

Kagan A, Harris BR, Winkelstein W *et al.* (1974). Epidemiological studies of coronary heart disease and stroke in Japanese men living in Japan, Hawaii, and California: demographic, physical, dietary, and biochemical characteristics. *J. Chron. Dis.*, **27**, 345–64.

Keys A (1975). Coronary heart disease—the global picture. *Atherosclerosis*, **22**, 149–92.

Kirby M (2008). Cholesterol targets: where will we be in 2008? *Ger. Med.*, **38**, 21–7.

LaRosa JC, Grundy SM, Waters DD *et al.* (2005). Intensive lipid lowering with atorvastatin in patients with stable coronary artery disease. *N. Engl. J. Med.*, **352**, 1425–35.

Lipid Research Clinics Program Epidemiology Committee (1979). Plasma lipid distributions in selected North American populations: the Lipid Clinics Program Prevalence Study. *Circulation*, **60**, 427–39.

Mann JI, Lewis B, Shepherd J *et al.* (1988). Blood lipid concentrations and other cardiovascular risk factors: distribution, prevalence, and detection in Britain. *Br. Med. J.*, **296**, 1702–6.

Multiple Risk Factor Intervention Trial study group. Multiple Risk Factor Intervention Trial (1982). *J. Am. Med. Assoc.*, **248**, 1465–77.

O'Keefe JH, Cordain L, Harris WH, Moe RM, and Vogel R (2004). Optimal low-density lipoprotein is 50 to 70 mg/dl. Lower is better and physiologically normal. *J. Am. Coll. Cardiol.*, **43**, 2142–6.

Stamler J, Daviglus ML, Garside DB *et al.* (2000). Relationship of baseline serum cholesterol levels in three large cohorts of younger men to long-term coronary, cardiovascular and all-cause mortality and to longevity. *J. Am. Med. Assoc.*, **284**, 311–8.

UK HDL-C Consensus Group (2004). Role of fibrates in reducing coronary risk: a UK consensus. *Curr. Med. Res. Opin.*, **20**, 241–7.

Willett WC, Green A, Stampfer MJ *et al.* (1987). Relative and absolute excess risks of coronary heart disease among women who smoke cigarettes. *N. Engl. J. Med.*, **317**, 1303–9.

Chapter 3

Lipid particles

Key points

- Lipids in the blood join with apoproteins to form soluble complexes.
- Lipid particles can be separated by mass, using an ultracentrifuge or by electrophoresis.
- In everyday use, levels of total cholesterol (TC), high-density lipoprotein cholesterol (HDL-C), and triglyceride (TG) are measured in an autoanalyser, and levels of low-density lipoprotein cholesterol (LDL-C) derived.

3.1 Introduction

Cholesterol is vital to body function, and TG fat is an important fuel source, delivering twice as much energy as carbohydrate. Both are present in serum, along with smaller amounts of phospholipids and free fatty acids. Cholesterol is in the form of free cholesterol or cholesterol esterified to fatty acids. The vast majority of serum lipids are present in particles known as lipoproteins, which also include proteins known as apolipoproteins.

The arrangement of lipids in lipoproteins follows a common pattern, with particles containing more hydrophobic lipids such as TGs and cholesterol esters in their core, with more hydrophilic lipids (free cholesterol and phospholipids) on the outside. The amount of lipid differs significantly between different particles, with the largest particles (chylomicrons) containing most lipid and the smallest particles (HDL) containing the least (Table 3.1).

In contrast, apolipoproteins differ between lipoprotein classes and determine the metabolic fate of lipoprotein particles by acting as receptor ligands or by activating or inhibiting enzymes involved in lipid metabolism (see Section 3.5 later).

3.2 Mass-based analysis

Separation of lipids by ultracentrifugation (Havel *et al.*, 1955) lead to the classification of lipid disorders endorsed by the WHO (Fredrickson *et al.*, 1967) (see Table 3.2). It is important to remember that this classification does not correlate well with the clinical picture, as the rarest disorder appears first. Separation by electrophoresis follows a similar pattern, as it too measures mass or density. The equivalent nomenclature is shown in Table 3.2 as well. More sophisticated ultracentrifugation has enabled LDL and HDL particles to be subdivided into at least three bands. Thus small dense LDL3 is more atherogenic than larger lighter LDL1. These methods are time consuming and are now rarely performed outside a reference laboratory.

Table 3.1 Lipid particles—size and composition			
Lipoprotein	Density (g/mL)	Mean particle diameter (nm)	Electrophoretic mobility
Chylomicrons	<0.95	500	Origin
Very low density lipoproteins (VLDL)	0.95–1.006	43	Pre-beta
Intermediate density lipoproteins (IDL)	1.006–1.019	27	Beta-1
Low-density lipoproteins (LDL)	1.019–1.063	22	Beta
High-density lipoproteins (HDL)	1.063–1.21	8	Alpha

Table 3.2 Frederickson's classification of lipid disorders			
Type	Name	Particle	Electrophoresis
I	Hyperchylomicronaemia	Chylos	Chylos
IIa	Familial hyper-cholesterolaemia (FH) or polygenic	LDL	β-lipoprotein
IIb	Familial combined hyperlipidaemia (FCH), mixed hyperlipidaemia	FCH, mixed hyperlipidaemia	β- and pre-β-lipoprotein
III	β- and pre-β-lipoprotein	IDL	Broad band
IV	Hypertriglyceridaemia	VLDL	Pre-β-lipoprotein
V	Severe mixed hyperlipidaemia	VLDL + Chylos	Pre-β-lipoprotein + chylos

3.3 **Compositional analysis**

The usual laboratory measurements are of TC, TG, and HDL, and then LDL can be derived from Friedewald's equation:

$$LDL\text{-}C = TC - HDL\text{-}C - TG/2.2$$

It should be noted that high TG values (>4 mmol/L) invalidate the equation. The ratio of TC:HDL-C or LDL-C:HDL-C is thought to be more informative than TC or LDL-C alone. The simplified classification shown in Table 3.3 is clinically relevant and in wide use.

Note that in Europe the lipid levels are expressed in mmol/L, whereas in the USA, mass units are used (mg/dL). To convert the mass units to molar, divide by 38.6 for cholesterol and 88.6 for TG, for example 240 mg/dL is 6.2 mmol/L. As an approximation divide by 40 and 90, respectively.

3.4 **Alimentary lipaemia**

Chylos and VLDL levels (TGs) rise after food (postprandial alimentary lipaemia) as the fat content of the meal is absorbed, so that the serum (or plasma) becomes turbid or cloudy. There is currently renewed interest in the prolonged area under the lipaemia curve that may be seen in diabetes and other conditions, and this may be a better indicator of risk than a single TG value alone.

To avoid confusion, TG levels should be measured after fasting for >12 h, whereas LDL and HDL particles remain stable after food. Always remember though that a lipid profile is at best a 'freeze-frame snapshot' of an ongoing dynamic metabolic process.

3.5 **Apolipoproteins**

The proteins attached to the various lipid particles are highly specific and are not just present to enhance aqueous solubility. Some (such as apolipoprotein (apo) B100 and E) are recognized by their respective receptors and hence initiate binding. Others (such as apo C-II) act as a co-factor for the degrading enzyme, in this case lipoprotein lipase. Defects in apolipoproteins may cause recognizable clinical problems, such as defective apo B100 can mimic FCH (Chapter 7) and subjects with apo E2/E2 isoforms may develop remnant hyperlipidaemia (Chapter 8).

Table 3.3 Simplified classification of lipid disorders
• Abnormal TC:HDL-C ratio
• Raised fasting TGs
• Mixed hyperlipidaemia

3.6 **Lipoprotein (a)**

This particle (Lp(a)) resembles LDL but contains both apo B100 and apo (a) (Table 3.4). This unique apolipoprotein bears a strong resemblance to plasminogen, and hence Lp(a) was thought to form a link between lipids and the coagulation system. Lp(a) contains folded proteins (called 'kringles' after the Danish pastry) and the large variability in molecular weight of Lp(a) (230–850 kDa) relates to the number of times kringle 4 is repeated. The physiological role of Lp(a) is unclear, as it is not present in many mammalian species, and low or absent levels do not seem to cause a problem. In man, the distribution of levels in the population is markedly skewed to the left. Low levels occur in liver disease, and levels can be reduced by nicotinic acid.

Table 3.4 Apolipoproteins and their function		
Apolipoprotein	**Main functions**	**Associated lipoprotein**
Apo AI	Ligand for HDL Co-factor for lecithin cholesterol acyltransferase (LCAT)	Chylomicrons, HDL
Apo AII	Ligand for HDL Co-factor for LCAT	Chylomicrons, HDL
Apo AIV	Ligand for HDL Activates LCAT	Chylomicrons, HDL
Apo (a)	Provides structural integrity for Lp(a)	Lp(a)
Apo B48	Provides structural integrity for chylomicrons	Chylomicrons
Apo B100	Provides structural integrity for VLDL, IDL, and LDL Ligand for LDL receptor	VLDL, IDL, LDL
Apo CI	Activates LCAT and lipoprotein lipase	Chylomicrons, VLDL, IDL, HDL
Apo CII	Activates LCAT and lipoprotein lipase	Chylomicrons, VLDL, IDL, HDL
Apo CIII	Inhibits lipoprotein lipase Inhibits hepatic lipase Modulates uptake by lipoprotein-related receptor (via binding to proteoglycans)	Chylomicrons, VLDL, IDL, HDL
Apo D	Unknown	HDL

Table 3.4 (Contd.)

Apolipoprotein	Main functions	Associated lipoprotein
Apo E	Ligand for apo B/E receptor	Chylomicrons, VLDL, IDL, LDL
	Ligand for apo E2 receptor	
	Ligand for lipoprotein-related receptor	
Apo J	Implicated in cell membrane protection	HDL

Originally, Lp(a) was thought to be a determinant of morbidity in FH (Seed *et al.*, 1990) but this has not been substantiated (Neil *et al.*, 2004). Levels may also be higher after coronary angioplasty (Desmarais *et al.*, 1995) or cardiac transplantation (Barbir *et al.*, 1992). A true role for this fascinating particle remains to be found.

Lp(a) should not be confused with lipoprotein-associated phospholipase (LP-PLA$_2$), a marker for inflammation (see Chapter 5).

References

Barbir M, Kushwaha S, Hunt B *et al.* (1992). Lipoprotein (a) and accelerated coronary artery disease in cardiac transplant recipients. *Lancet*, **340**, 1500–02.

Desmarais RL, Sarembock IJ, Ayers CR *et al.* (1995). Elevated lipoprotein (a) is a risk factor for clinical recurrence after coronary balloon angioplasty. *Circulation*, **91**, 1403–9.

Fredrickson DS, Levy RI, and Lees RS (1967). Fat transport in lipoproteins—an integrated approach to mechanisms and disorders. *N. Engl. J. Med.*, **276**, 34–42, 94–103, 148–56, 215–25, 273–81.

Havel RJ, Eder HA, and Bragdon JH (1955). The determination and chemical composition of ultracentrifugally separated lipoproteins in human serum. *J. Clin. Invest.*, **34**, 1345–53.

Neil HAW, Seagroatt V, Betteridge DJ *et al.* (2004). Established and emerging coronary risk factors in patients with heterozygous familial hypercholesterolaemia. *Heart*, **90**, 1431–7.

Seed M, Hopplicher F, Reaveley D *et al.* (1990). Relation of serum lipoprotein (a) concentration and apolipoprotein (a) phenotype to coronary heart disease in patients with familial hypercholesterolemia. *N. Engl. J. Med.*, **322**, 1494–9.

Chapter 4

Lipid metabolism

Key points

- Lipid particles from food are transported in the blood as triglyceride (TG) and chylomicrons for use as muscle fuel or for storage, and the remaining particles are cleared by the liver.
- The liver can synthesize TGs and cholesterol during periods of fasting.
- Reverse cholesterol transport utilizes high-density lipoprotein cholesterol (HDL-C).

Lipid metabolism can be considered under three main headings: the exogenous pathway, the endogenous pathway, and reverse cholesterol transport.

4.1 Exogenous lipid metabolism

Exogenous lipid metabolism describes the process by which lipids from the diet are absorbed and used within the body. Dietary lipids are absorbed by the mucosal cells of the intestine which re-esterify cholesterol and free fatty acids to produce TGs and cholesterol esters. These lipids, along with phospholipids and unesterified cholesterol, are packaged together with apo B48 to form the largest triglyceride-rich lipoproteins, chylomicrons. Chylomicrons are characterized by the presence of apo B48, which is a low molecular weight form of apo B100. This apoprotein is specifically produced by the intestine (Guo, 2005) and only contains residues 1–2152 (48% of apo B100), thus preventing chylomicrons from interacting with the LDL receptor.

Newly formed chylomicrons are rapidly metabolized to chylomicron remnants following their secretion into the general circulation. An exchange of apoproteins occurs between chylomicrons and HDL, and the chylomicron remnants acquire C and E apoproteins in exchange for apo A proteins. Chylomicron remnants become relatively deplete in TGs due to the hydrolysis of the particles' TG core by lipoprotein lipase, an enzyme which is anchored to the endothelium. In addition, cholesterol ester is transferred from mature HDL to the chylomicron remnants in exchange for TG by cholesteryl ester transfer protein (CETP) (de Grooth et al., 2004). The remaining chylomicron remnants are rapidly cleared from the circulation by hepatic receptors specific for apo E.

The exogenous pathway efficiently delivers TG to skeletal muscle and adipose tissue and deposits cholesterol for processing in the liver. Following the ingestion of food, chylomicrons are normally undetectable following a 12-h fast, allowing baseline TG measurement.

4.2 Endogenous lipid metabolism

Endogenous lipid metabolism describes the process by which the liver produces TG-rich particles and releases them into the circulation during periods of fasting. Fatty acids surplus to oxidative requirements are utilized by the liver for the synthesis of TG and phospholipid. Cholesterol can also be produced endogenously by a pathway which includes the rate-limiting enzyme β-hydroxy-β-methylglutaryl-coenzyme A reductase (HMG-CoA reductase), which is subject to inhibition by the end product, cholesterol. Although the liver has the capacity to synthesize cholesterol and TG, it is more efficient to utilize preformed lipids derived from the diet or excess stores in adipose tissue.

In the fasting (post-absorptive) state, very low density lipoprotein (VLDL) replaces chylomicrons as the most abundant TG-rich lipoprotein and the metabolism of VLDL is similar to that of chylomicrons (Gibbons et al., 2004). The liver packages TG, cholesterol, cholesterol ester, and phospholipid together with C apoproteins, apo B100, and apo E form nascent (newly formed) VLDL, which is secreted into the bloodstream. Similar to chylomicrons, nascent VLDL becomes relatively deplete in TGs following its interaction with lipoprotein lipase and CETP. The particle also sheds apo C and E proteins to produce a 'VLDL remnant' known as intermediate density lipoprotein (IDL). Unlike chylomicron remnants, IDL can be taken up by the liver or may undergo further delipidation and loss of apoproteins to yield LDL.

The VLDL class encompasses an extremely heterogeneous population of lipoprotein particles that differ in size (80 to 1200 nm), composition, and metabolic fate. Large buoyant VLDL tends to be metabolized to IDL, which is subsequently cleared via apo B/E receptor-mediated uptake in the liver. Conversely, smaller VLDL particles complete the metabolic cascade by producing IDL, which ultimately yields LDL. LDL is removed by apo B100 receptor-mediated uptake in the liver, although LDL can also be utilized by extrahepatic tissue to provide cholesterol for normal cellular functions.

4.3 **Reverse cholesterol transport**

Reverse cholesterol transport describes the process by which HDL particles pick up cholesterol from the arterial wall and transport it back to the liver, where it is excreted in bile (von Eckardstein et al., 2005). The HDL lipoproteins (see Chapter 3) are the smallest and most dense lipid particles, and can be divided into two subclasses (HDL2 which are larger and HDL3 which are smaller and more dense). Plasma concentrations of the HDL3 subclass are more abundant than HDL2 (3:1). The major apoprotein constituents of HDL are the A apoproteins (AI, AII, AIV; see Table 3.4) and these are responsible for modulating HDL metabolism. The A apoproteins function as acceptors of cellular cholesterol, serve as co-factors for lecithin cholesterol acyl transferase (LCAT), and act as ligands for HDL receptors.

The liver and intestine synthesize and secrete nascent, discoid HDL, which consists mainly of apo E, apo C's, phospholipid, and free cholesterol. The particle acquires apo A proteins which provides the lipoprotein with the capacity to utilize LCAT and adenosine triphosphate-binding cassette protein A1 (ABCA-1). The ABCA-1 transporter protein facilitates the efflux of intracellular cholesterol through an interaction with apo AI on lipid-deplete HDL (Fielding and Fielding, 2001). Following this, LCAT catalyses the esterification of HDL cholesterol, and the hydrophobicity of the sterol-ester results in its relocation from the surface of the lipoprotein to the hydrophobic core of the particle. The surface of HDL is available to accept more free cholesterol, forming mature spherical HDL particles.

Cholesterol can be transferred out of HDL to TG-rich lipoproteins by the action of CETP. Inhibition of CETP could therefore increase circulating HDL-C levels, with a beneficial effect on CV risk (see Chapter 9). In fact, the situation is more complex (Dullaart et al., 2007) and the clinical value of CETP inhibition remains to be proven.

HDL-C not only is involved in reverse cholesterol transport but also has many other functions. HDL particles are antioxidant, anti-inflammatory, anti-thrombotic and may stabilize endothelial function (O'Connell and Genest, 2001). Therefore HDL-C particles are cardioprotective, and conversely, low HDL-C levels are potentially atherogenic (Barter and Rye, 1996; Assmann and Nofer, 2003).

References

Assmann G and Nofer J-R (2003). Atheroprotective effects of high-density lipoproteins. Ann. Rev. Med., **54**, 321–41.

Barter PJ and Rye K-A (1996). High density lipoproteins and coronary heart disease. Atherosclerosis, **121**, 1–12.

Dullaart RPF, Dallinga-Thie GM, Wolffenbuttel BHR, and van Tol A (2007). CETP inhibition in cardiovascular risk management: a critical appraisal. *Eur. J. Clin. Invest.*, **37**, 90–8.

Eckardstein von A, Hersberger M, and Rohrer L (2005). Current understanding of the metabolism and biological actions of HDL. *Curr. Opin. Clin. Nutr. Metab. Care*, **8**: 147–52.

Fielding CJ and Fielding PE (1995). Molecular physiology of reverse cholesterol transport. *J. Lipid Res.*, **36**: 211–28.

Gibbons GF, Wiggins D, Brown A-M, and Hebbachi A-M (2004). Synthesis and function of hepatic very-low-density lipoprotein. *Biochem. Soc. Trans.*, **32**: 59–64.

Grooth de G, Klerkx AHEM, Stroes ESG, Stalenhoef AFH, Kastelein JJP, and Kuivenhoven JA. (2004). A review of CETP and its relation to atherosclerosis. *J. Lipid Res.*, **45**: 1967–74.

Guo Q, Avramoghu RK, and Adeli K (2005). Intestinal assembly and secretion of highly dense/lipid poor apolipoprotein B48-containing lipoprotein particles in the fasting state: evidence for induction by insulin resistance and exogenous fatty acids. *Metabolism*, **54**: 689–97.

O'Connell BJ and Genest J Jr. (2001). High-density lipoproteins and endothelial function. *Circulation*, **104**, 1978–83.

Chapter 5

Mechanisms of atherogenesis

Key points
• Atherosclerosis is caused by lipid deposition and inflammation in the arterial wall.
• Native low-density lipoprotein (LDL) is atherogenic when modified, for example by oxidation.
• Unstable plaques may rupture and cause acute thrombotic occlusion.
• Lipid-lowering treatment can reduce plaque size and increase stability.

There is now widespread acceptance that two key processes drive the development of atherosclerosis—lipid deposition and inflammation within the arterial wall. All of the well-recognized risk factors for atherosclerosis contribute to the process by influencing one or both of these mechanisms.

5.1 Lipid deposition

The earliest stage of atherosclerosis—the fatty streak (Ross, 1993)—is detectable from early childhood in individuals brought up in Western society (Stary, 1989). The first stage of the atherosclerotic process is characterized by lipid transport into the arterial wall, where excess lipid begins to accumulate. Since most cholesterol in the blood is contained within LDL particles, LDL is the chief source of lipid deposits. LDL particles are retained in the arterial wall as a result of interactions with connective tissue components such as proteoglycans and collagen, and it is likely that retention is a more important process than transport of LDL into the arterial wall.

Within the arterial wall, LDL particles interact with cells and become modified, mainly as a result of oxidation of lipids and proteins within the lipoprotein particles (Steinberg et al., 1989; Witztum, 1994; Berliner and Watson, 2005). Oxidized LDL particles are taken up by macrophages and smooth muscle cells in an uncontrolled way, and excess lipid accumulating in the cells transforms them into foam cells, which are a characteristic feature of the atherosclerotic plaque (Figure 5.1).

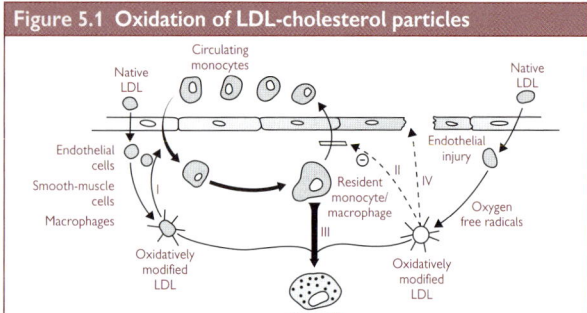

Figure 5.1 Oxidation of LDL-cholesterol particles

As the atherosclerotic plaque grows, it is characterized by a soft lipid core surrounded by inflammatory cells and covered by a fibrous cap. Initially, the plaque grows within the arterial wall, but as time goes on it may gradually intrude on the lumen which becomes narrowed and results in a restriction of blood flow. Plaques which contain large amounts of lipid and inflammatory cells are more unstable, meaning that the fibrous cap is thinner and more liable to rupture, which exposes the soft lipid core to the circulating blood. If this occurs, a thrombus may form and expand rapidly to completely occlude the arterial lumen, precipitating a myocardial infarction or stroke (Falk et al., 1995). Aggressive lipid management in patients with established atherosclerotic lesions can reduce the size of the soft lipid core and reduce inflammation in the plaque. This will result in a more stable lesion and therefore a reduced risk of cardiovascular complications.

5.2 Inflammation

Oxidized LDL is also a potent inducer of the inflammatory process, and is largely responsible for the recruitment and retention of inflammatory cells into the atherosclerotic plaque. Once present, inflammatory cells produce a range of mediators which encourage proliferation of cells within the plaque and render the growing plaque more unstable and prone to rupture (Sattar et al., 2003; Packard and Libby, 2008). Raised levels of C-reactive protein (CRP) act as a marker for inflammation, and are raised in patients with coronary artery disease. Furthermore, their reduction, for example with statins is associated with an improved outcome (Nissen et al., 2005; Ridker et al., 2008). Lipoprotein-associated phospholipase (Lp-PLA$_2$) is another marker for inflammation, independent of CRP (Ballantyne et al., 2004).

Figure 5.1 is reproduced with permission from Quinn M, Parthasarathy S, Fong LG, and Steinberg D. (1987). Oxidatively modified low density lipoproteins: A potential role in recruitment and retention of monocyte/macrophages during atherogenesis. PNAS, **84**(9): 2995–8.

5.3 **Assessment of vascular disease**

Using coronary angiography, it is possible to demonstrate reduced progression of coronary artery lesions with lipid-lowering therapy (Watts *et al.*, 1992) or even regression of existing lesions (Brown *et al.*, 1990; MAAS Investigators, 1994). However, such methods are invasive and hard to justify for research purposes only. There has therefore been much interest in non-invasive surrogate markers for atherosclerosis.

Endothelial dysfunction can be identified at an early stage in the atherosclerotic process, before anatomical changes are apparent (Creager *et al.*, 1990; Zeiher *et al.*, 1991; Celermajer *et al.*, 1992; Sorensen *et al.*, 1994), and is potentially reversible (Stroes *et al.*, 1995). Endothelial function can be assessed by forearm blood flow or by the more sophisticated flow-mediated dilation. In addition, the pulse waveform and analysis of reflected waveforms give an index of arterial stiffness.

The intima:media thickness ratio in the carotid artery can be directly measured by ultrasound (Blankenhorn *et al.*, 1993), and used to demonstrate early pathology (Wiegman *et al.*, 2004). It can also be used (with less success) as an end point in clinical trials (Kastelein *et al.*, 2008; Stein, 2008). Intravascular ultrasound can be used in the coronary arteries (Nissen *et al.*, 2005).

More recently, magnetic resonance imaging (MRI) has been used to identify endothelial dysfunction (Sorensen *et al.*, 2002), fibrous cap rupture (Yuan *et al.*, 2002), or thrombosis (Moody *et al.*, 2003).

5.4 **Other lipids**

The processes outlined earlier are driven mainly by LDL particles, but are also promoted by triglyceride-rich lipoproteins such as VLDL and IDL. In contrast, the HDL inhibits the process of atherogenesis by promoting the removal of excess lipid from the arterial wall and as a result of its antioxidant and anti-inflammatory properties (Ansell *et al.*, 2007).

5.5 **Conclusion**

As can be seen, therefore, the two processes which characterize atherosclerosis are both dependent on excess lipid, particularly in the form of LDL cholesterol. Therefore, effective management of serum lipids is a powerful strategy to prevent the development of atherosclerosis.

References

Ansell BJ, Fonarow GC, and Fogelman AM (2007). The paradox of dysfunctional high-density lipoprotein. *Curr. Opin. Lipidol.*, **18**, 427–34.

Ballantyne CM, Hoogeveen RC, Bang H, *et al.* (2004). Lipoprotein-associated phospholipase A_2, high-sensitivity C-reactive protein, and risk for incident coronary heart disease in middle-aged men and women in the Atherosclerosis Risk in Communities (ARIC) study. *Circulation*, **109**: 837–42.

Berliner JA and Watson AD (2005). A role for oxidized phospholipids in atherosclerosis. *N. Engl. J. Med.*, **353**, 9–11; 1869.

Blankenhorn DH, Selzer RH, Crawford DW *et al.* (1993). Beneficial effects of colestipol–niacin therapy on the common carotid artery. *Circulation*, **88**, 20–8.

Brown G, Albers JJ, Fisher LD *et al.* (1990). Regression of coronary artery disease as a result of intensive lipid-lowering therapy in men with high levels of apolipoprotein B. *N. Engl. J. Med.*, **323**, 1289–98.

Celermajer DS, Sorensen KE, Gooch VM *et al.* (1992). Non-invasive detection of endothelial dysfunction in children and adults at risk of atherosclerosis. *Lancet*, **340**, 1111–5.

Creager MA, Cooke JP, Mendelsohn ME *et al.* (1990). Impaired vasodilation of forearm resistance vessels in hypercholesterolemic humans. *J. Clin. Invest.*, **86**, 228–34.

Falk E, Shah PK, and Fuster V (1995). Coronary plaque disruption. *Circulation*, **92**, 657–71.

Kastelein JJP, Akdim F, Stroes ESG *et al.* (2008). Simvastatin with or without ezetimibe in familial hypercholesterolemia (ENHANCE). *N. Engl. J. Med.*, **358**, 1431–43.

MAAS Investigators (1994). Effect of simvastatin on coronary atheroma: the Multicentre Anti-Atheroma Study (MAAS). *Lancet*, **344**, 633–8.

Moody AR, Murphy RE, Morgan PS *et al.* (2003). Characterization of complicated carotid plaque with magnetic resonance direct thrombus imaging on patients with cerebral ischemia, *Circulation*, **107**, 3047–52.

Nissen SE, Tuzcu EM, Schoenhagen P *et al.* (2005). Statin treatment, LDL cholesterol, C-reactive protein, and coronary artery disease. *N. Engl. J. Med.*, **352**, 29–38.

Packard RR and Libby P (2008). Inflammation in atherosclerosis: from vascular biology to biomarker discovery and risk prediction. *Clin. Chem.*, **54**, 24–38.

Ross R (1993). The pathogenesis of atherosclerosis: a perspective for the 1990s. *Nature*, **362**, 801–9.

Ridker PM, Danielson E, Francisco AH, *et al.* (2008). Rosuvastatin to prevent vascular events in men and women with elevated C-reactive protein. *N. Engl. J. Med.*, **359**: 2195–207.

Sattar N, McCarey DW, Capell H *et al.* (2003). Explaining how "high-grade" systemic inflammation accelerates vascular risk in rheumatoid arthritis. *Circulation*, **108**, 2957–63.

Sorensen KE, Celemajer DS, Georgakopoulos D, Hatcher G, Betteridge DJ, and Deanfield JE (1994). Impairment of endothelium-dependent dilation is an early event in children with familial hypercholesterolemia and is related to the Lipoprotein (a) level. *J. Clin. Invest.*, **93**, 50–5.

Sorensen MB, Collins P, Ong PJL *et al.* (2002). Long-term use of contraceptive depot medroxyprogesterone acetate in young women impairs arterial endothelial function assessed by cardiovascular magnetic resonance. *Circulation*, **106**, 1646–51.

Stary HC (1989). Evolution and progression of atherosclerotic lesions in coronary arteries of children and young adults. *Arteriosclerosis*, **9**, I-19–I-32.

Stein EA (2008). Additional lipid lowering trials using surrogate measurement of atherosclerosis by carotid intima-media thickness: more clarity or confusion? *J. Am. Coll. Cardiol.*, **52**: 2120–3.

Steinberg D, Parthasarathy S, Carew TE, Khoo JC, and Witzum JL (1989). Beyond cholesterol. Modifications of low-density lipoprotein that increase its atherogenicity. *New Engl. J. Med.*, **320**, 915–24.

Stroes ESG, Koomans HA, de Bruijn TWA, and Rabelink TJ (1995). Vascular function in the forearm of hypercholesterolaemic patients off and on lipid-lowering medication. *Lancet*, **346**, 467–71.

Watts GF, Lewis B, Brunt JNH *et al.* (1992). Effects on coronary artery disease of lipid-lowering diet, or diet plus cholestyramine, in the St. Thomas' Atherosclerosis Regression Study (STARS). *Lancet*, **339**, 563–9.

Wiegman A, de Groot E, Hutten BA *et al.* (2004). Arterial intima:media thickness in childhood. A study in familial hypercholesterolaemia heterozygotes and their siblings. *Lancet*, **363**, 368–70.

Witztum J (1994). The oxidation hypothesis of atherosclerosis. *Lancet*, **344**, 793–5.

Yuan C, Zhang S-X, Polissar NL *et al.* (2002). Identification of fibrous cap rupture with magnetic resonance imaging is highly associated with recent transient ischemic attack or stroke. *Circulation*, **105**, 181–5.

Zeiher AM, Drexler H, Wollschläger H, and Just H (1991). Modulation of coronary vasomotor control in humans. *Circulation*, **83**, 391–401.

Chapter 6

Hypercholesterolaemia and risk assessment

Key points

- In patients with established vascular disease or very high risk (secondary prevention), the aim should be to reduce total cholesterol (TC) to <5 mmol/L and low-density lipoprotein cholesterol (LDL-C) to <3 mmol/L.
- Ideal levels are TC <4 mmol/L and LDL-C <2 mmol/L, but these may not be achievable in everybody.
- In patients with no known vascular disease (primary prevention), the decision to treat depends on the individual's risk profile, but the targets are the same.
- A holistic approach includes assessment of other risk factors as well, such as hypertension, smoking, diabetes, or obesity.

6.1 Primary prevention

Primary prevention refers to the treatment of cholesterol levels in asymptomatic individuals with no history of vascular disease. The debate about normal, usual, prevalent, or desirable levels of TC in the population has been considered earlier (Chapter 3), but in an individual, the decision to treat the lipid profile depends on their risk of developing a major cardiovascular event over the next 10 yrs (JBS2, 2005). A probability of <10% is low risk, 10%–20% intermediate risk, and >20% high risk. High-risk individuals should be treated.

In addition to the lipid levels (TC, LDL-C and HDL-C), calculation of risk involves age, sex, and other factors such as hypertension or cigarette smoking. Risk can be assessed using a computer algorithm. A number of such algorithms are available, generally based on large population studies. The JBS guidelines (JBS, 2005), reprinted in the British National Formulary, are based on the Framingham study. The risk scores are shown in Figures 6.1 (men) and 6.2 (women). Numerous other bodies including the European Society for Cardiology (ESC) (Graham et al., 2007) and the Food and Drug Administration (FDA) in the USA (Expert Panel Report, 2001) have also given broadly similar recommendations but in the interests of simplicity we have not included these.

Figure 6.1 JBS risk chart for primary prevention in men

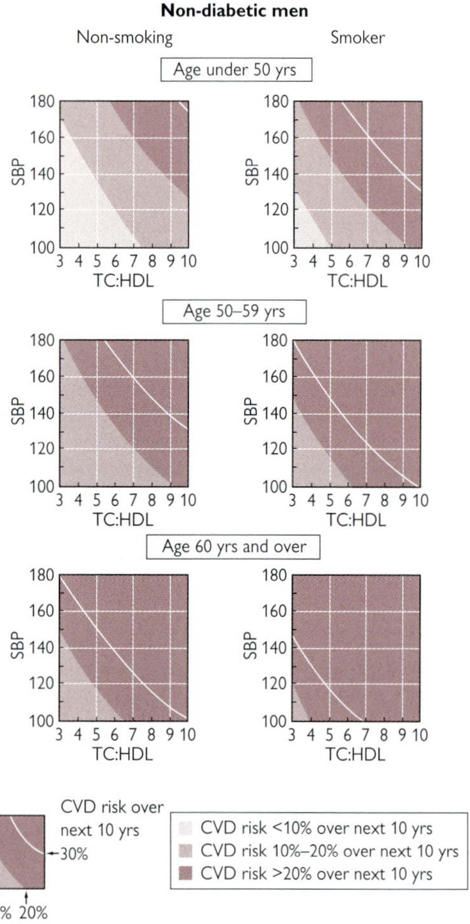

Non-diabetic men
Non-smoking
Smoker
Age under 50 yrs
Age 50–59 yrs
Age 60 yrs and over
SBP
180
160
140
120
100
3 4 5 6 7 8 9 10
TC:HDL
CVD risk over next 10 yrs
30%
10% 20%
CVD risk <10% over next 10 yrs
CVD risk 10%–20% over next 10 yrs
CVD risk >20% over next 10 yrs

SBP = systolic blood pressure, mmHg
TC:HDL = serum total cholesterol to HDL-cholesterol ratio

⚠ These charts are not appropriate for use with patients with pre-existing CHD, FH, chronic renal dysfunction, or diabetes.

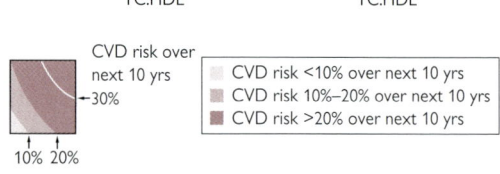

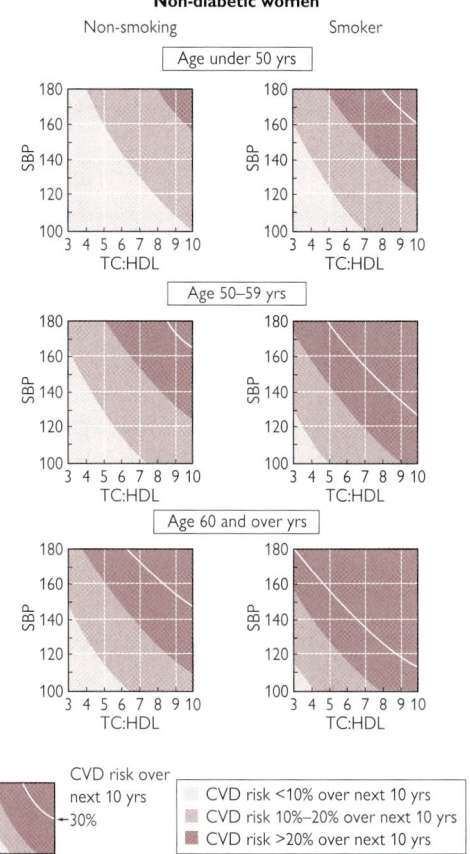

Figure 6.2 JBS risk chart for primary prevention in women

Figure 6.2 is reproduced with permission from Professor P. Durrington, © the University of Manchester, UK.

In general, women with no additional risk factors tend to be at low risk, and as a consequence the benefits of treatment are small. It can also be seen that given the cholesterol distribution in Western Europe, a significant proportion of the population could qualify for treatment, which has major ethical and financial implications.

One of the problems with risk tables and algorithms is that they fail to take account of all risk factors, and therefore may underestimate risk in certain groups of patients. For instance, South Asians, those with renal failure, those with vascular inflammation, or those with a notable family history of premature cardiovascular disease are likely to have their risk significantly underestimated. In the presence of such additional risk factors, it is pragmatic to multiply up the estimate produced by the algorithm or table by 1.3 to 1.5 for each additional factor. UK guidelines for risk assessment and the treatment of lipid disorders have recently been published (NICE, 2008).

6.2 **Secondary prevention**

In patients with known vascular disease, risk has become reality. The risk equations do not apply, and nearly everyone qualifies for treatment. Patients with diabetes, severe hypertension, or heterozygous familial hypercholesterolaemia (HeFH)/familial combined hyperlipidaemia (FCH) also belong to this category because of their marked propensity to develop premature coronary heart disease (CHD). Women in this category should be treated the same as men (see treating to new targets (TNT) trial, Chapter 12). We have added severe hypertriglyceridaemia to this list (Table 6.1) because of the risk of acute pancreatitis (see Chapter 8).

6.3 **Treatment targets**

There has been, and continues to be, considerable debate about appropriate therapeutic goals in the management of hyperlipidaemia. One approach is to have a single set of targets in all patients once a decision is made to commence treatment, and this is the approach recommended by the JBS (JBS, 2005; Table 6.2). For many patients

Table 6.1 **JBS recommendations for treatment**
Known vascular disease
Diabetes (type 1 or 2)
Hypertension with target organ damage
HeFH, FCH
Risk of CHD >20% over next 10 yrs
TC:high-density lipoprotein cholesterol (HDL-C) ratio >6
[Fasting triglyceride (TG) >10 mmol/L]

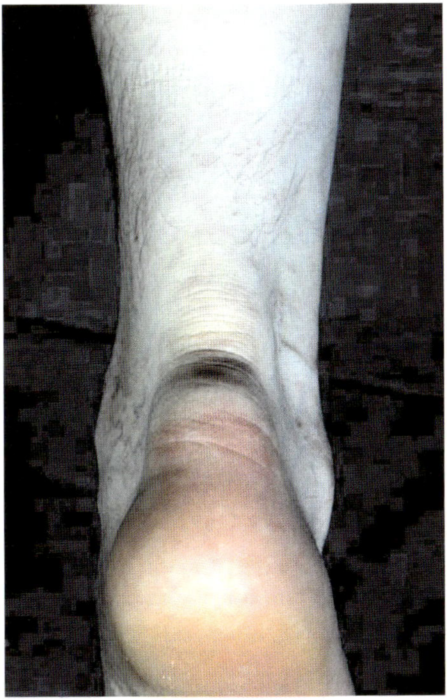

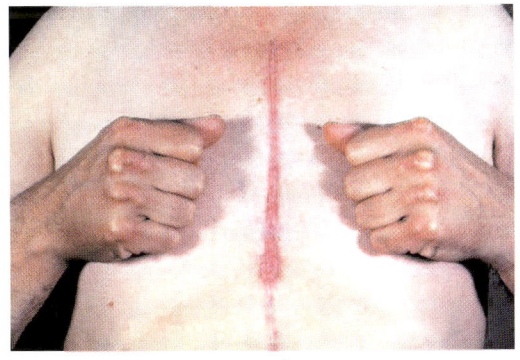

Plate 1 Achilles tendon thickening in a patient with FH

Plate 2 Scar from coronary artery surgery and tendon xanthomata in a patient with FH

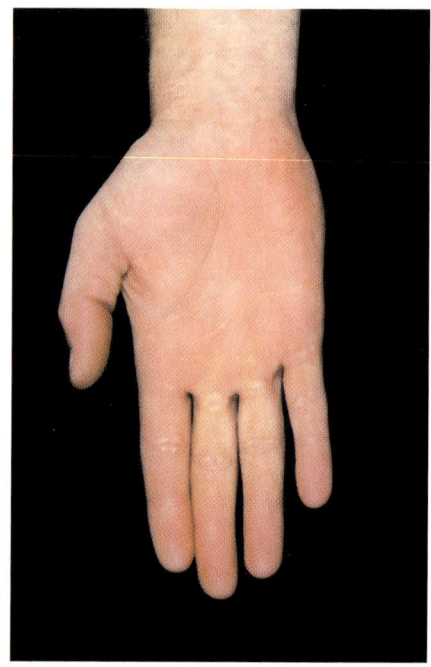

Plate 3 Palmar crease xanthomata in remnant (type III) dyslipidaemia

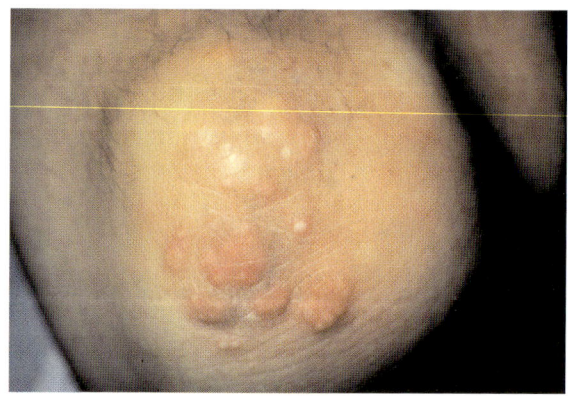

Plate 4 Tuberoeruptive xanthomata on the elbow of a patient with remnant (type III) hyperlipidaemia

Table 6.2 JBS targets for treatment
TC <4 mmol/L
LDL-C <2 mmol/L
HDL-C >1 mmol/L [males] or 1.2 mmol/L [females]
TG <1.7 mmol/L
Non-HDL-C <3 mmol/L

though a TC of <4 mmol/l and an LDL-C of <2 mmol/l remains a desirable goal rather than a practical reality, especially if the initial TC was >8 mmol/l, as may occur in FH (Chapter 7). For this reason, in the UK it is often suggested that the audit target should be TC <5 mmol/l and LDL-C <3 mmol/l.

Whilst this approach has the advantage of simplicity, some have argued that it lacks sufficient supporting evidence. An alternative approach therefore is to use differential therapeutic targets, with the lower levels used for those at highest risk, that is those patients with established vascular disease or diabetes. This is the recommended approach in the UK (NICE, 2008), and a similar approach is recommended in the USA, except that the target for LDL-C is lower at <1.8 mmol/l.

Most guidelines refer to targets for TC or LDL-C rather than HDL-C or TG, probably because of the lack of direct clinical trial evidence for interventions which target the latter, although such studies are currently under way. However, targets for HDL-C and TG have also been set (JBS, 2005; Table 6.2)'.

References

Expert Panel on detection, evaluation, and treatment of high blood cholesterol in adults: Executive Summary of the Third Report of the National Cholesterol Education Program (NCEP) (2001). J. Am. Med. Assoc., 285, 2486–97.

Graham I, Atar D, Borch-Johnsen K et al. (2007). European guidelines on cardiovascular disease prevention in clinical practice: executive summary. Atherosclerosis, 194, 1–45.

JBS2 (2005). Joint British Societies' Guidelines on prevention of cardiovascular disease in clinical practice. Heart, 91 (Suppl. V), 1–52.

National Institute for Health and Clinical Excellance (NICE) (2008). *Cardiovascular risk assessment, and the modification of blood lipids for the primary and secondary prevention of cardiovascular disease.* www.nice.org.uk/CG067

Chapter 7

Familial hypercholesterolaemia

> **Key points**
> - Heterozygous familial hypercholesterolaemia (HeFH) affects 1 in 500 of the population.
> - Levels of total cholesterol (TC) and low-density lipoprotein cholesterol (LDL-C) are approximately twice normal.
> - Inheritance is autosomal dominant.
> - In most families, the disorder is highly atherogenic.
> - Cascade screening from known affected individuals is strongly recommended.
> - Patients should be referred to a Lipid Clinic.

7.1 Introduction

In familial hypercholesterolaemia (FH), elevated levels of LDL-C are inherited in an autosomal codominant pattern. The clinical association of tendon xanthomata (TX) and high blood cholesterol levels was described many years ago (Burns, 1920) and the genetic basis for the disorder was described by Goldstein and Brown in 1975. HeFH occurs in about 1/500 of the population. The diagnostic criteria are shown in Table 7.1 (Scientific Steering Committee, 1999). A new diagnostic scoring system has also been proposed from Holland (Defesche, 2000; Table 7.2) and validated in Denmark (Damgaard et al., 2005).

Cholesterol levels rise to about twice normal due to a defect in LDL clearance, and affected individuals are at higher risk of developing premature coronary heart disease (CHD) than unaffected individuals (Slack, 1969). Untreated males aged 20–40 yrs are almost 100 times more likely to develop premature CHD (Betteridge et al., 1991).

HeFH is widespread throughout the world, but is more common in certain areas such as South Africa or French Canada, where the prevalence may reach 1/50. In addition, areas in which consanguineous marriages are permitted have a higher incidence of HeFH and therefore the chances of developing homozygous FH (HoFH) are increased (see below). HoFH is rare but fatal in childhood or adolescence if untreated.

Guidelines for the diagnosis and management of HeFH have been published recently (National Institute for Health and Clinical Excellence, 2008; Wierzbicki et al., 2008).

Table 7.1 Simon Broome Trust diagnostic criteria for FH
Definite FH = TC > 7.5 mmol/L (LDL-C 4.9) in adults, or
OR
TC > 6.7 mmol/L in children < 16 yrs old
AND
TX in the patient, or a first- or second-degree relative
OR
Defined genetic defect in the LDL-R or apo B-encoding genes
Possible FH = TC or LDL-C levels as above
AND
History of myocardial infarction (MI) at age <60 yrs in a first-degree relative
OR
History of MI at age <50 yrs in a second-degree relative
OR
TC >7.5 mmol/L in a first- or second-degree relative

Table 7.2 Dutch scoring system for the diagnosis of FH	
• Patient has premature CHD	2
• Patient has premature cerebral or peripheral vascular disease	1
• Patient has TX	6
• Patient has corneal arcus when aged <45 yrs	4
• First-degree relative with premature vascular disease	1
• First-degree relative with LDL-C >95th centile	
AND	
First-degree relative with TX or corneal arcus	
OR	
• Children <18 yrs with LDL-C >95th centile	2
• LDL-C > 8.5 mmol/L	8
• LDL-C 6.5–8.4 mmol/L	5
• LDL-C 5.0–6.4 mmol/L	3
• LDL-C 4.0–4.9 mmol/L	1
• Defined functional gene mutation	8
Premature = males < 55 yrs, females <60 yrs	
Definite FH = score 9 or more	
Probable FH = 6–8	
Possible FH = 3–5	

7.2 Clinical features

The main clinical problem relates to the inappropriately high level of circulating atherogenic LDL-C (see Chapter 5). Untreated, the burden of premature CHD becomes so high that at one time up to 5% of Coronary Care Unit admissions were thought to relate to HeFH. The only external sign is TX (see Figures 7.1–7.2), usually on the back of the hand, the Achilles tendon, or the patellar tendon. They are more common as age increases. Other signs such as xanthalesmata around the eyes or corneal arcus are not specific for HeFH. The combination of TX and high cholesterol levels in first-degree relatives enables the diagnosis of HeFH to be made. More recently the presence of a known gene defect can be used as evidence instead, and this has revealed that many families do not have TX.

> **Figure 7.1 Achilles tendon thickening in a patient with FH (see also Colour plate 1)**

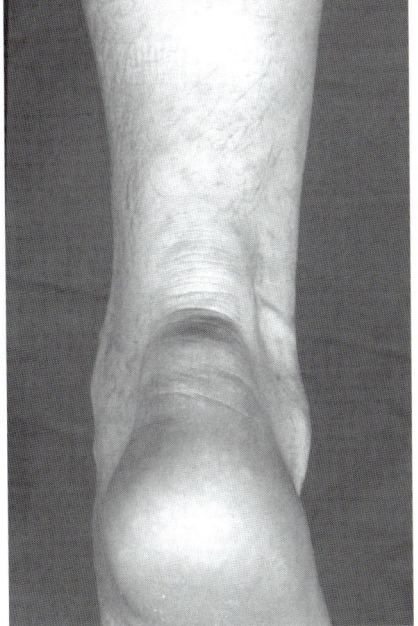

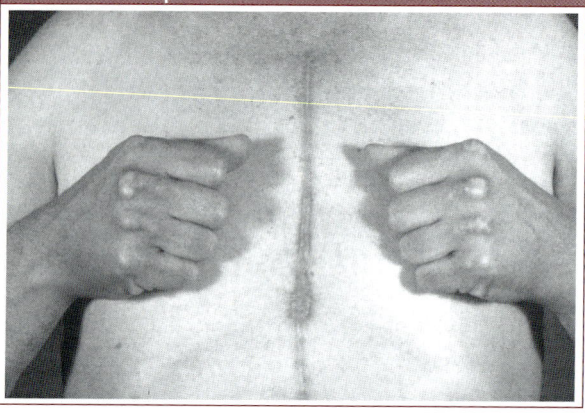

Figure 7.2 Scar from coronary artery surgery and tendon xanthomata in a patient with FH

7.3 **Genetics of FH**

The inheritance pattern is autosomal codominant, so males and females are affected equally. An affected individual (heterozygote) will pass the trait on to one in two of their children, whereas an unaffected individual can never pass it on. In the majority of families the problem arises in the gene for the LDL clearance receptor, encoded on chromosome 19q. The gene has 18 exons with intervening introns, and so far over 1600 mutations have been registered on the Website (http://www.ucl.ac.uk/fh; http://www.umd.necker.fr). In 10%–15% of cases the fault lies with the ligand for the LDL receptor, apolipoprotein B (familial dysbetalipoproteinaemia, FDB), which is phenotypically identical to HeFH (Tybjaerg-Hansen and Humphries, 1992). Other genes have been implicated rarely (Garcia *et al.*, 2001; Abifadel *et al.*, 2003).

The causal mutation differs from one family to another. In families with definite (TX positive) HeFH, the gene defect can be identified in >90%, whereas without TX, the rate falls to about 30% (Graham *et al.*, 2005; Tosi *et al.*, 2007).

7.4 **Prognosis of HeFH**

The first survey of the Simon Broome Association in Oxford indicated that men aged 20–40 were almost 100 times more likely to develop premature CHD than age-matched controls (Betteridge *et al.*, 1991). This is in contrast to other established risk factors for CHD such as smoking, which increases risk twofold, and diabetes (four-fold). It is interesting that the data for this survey were collected at a time when effective treatment (statins) was not available. Clearly it is unethical to conduct a long-term trial of active treatment vs placebo in HeFH, but a second survey some years later (Scientific Steering Committee, 1999) showed a reduction in events following the intro-duction of more modern treatments. More recently, the same group (Neil *et al.*, 2005) has confirmed the earlier finding (Mohrschladt *et al.*, 2004) that overall mortality in treated FH is similar to that in the general population. The rate of coronary disease remains higher than normal, but this appears to be balanced by a reduction in cancers, so that life insurance or mortgage terms should not be loaded if good control can be demonstrated.

A further detailed survey of potential interacting factors in the prognosis of patients with HeFH included other atherogenic factors such as Lp(a) and homocysteine (Neil *et al.*, 2004) and showed that only cigarette smoking clearly added to the risk, and this should therefore be strongly discouraged in patients with HeFH.

It is clear though that there is considerable variation in the severity of CHD between families and even within them (Kotze *et al.*, 1993; Sijbrands *et al.*, 2001). In view of this, the family history should be taken in to account when making treatment decisions, especially in children.

7.5 **Children with FH**

Children with HeFH have no signs or symptoms and so the abnor-mality can only be detected by screening (Nicholls, 2006). Clearly random screening of the whole population would not be cost effec-tive, as in any given primary school, only one or two children would be affected. Screening therefore follows from relatives of a known affected individual (proband) in a 'cascade' pattern (Department of Health, 2003; DeMott *et al.*, 2008). Ideally genotype should be used as it is specific, but the test is not yet widely available and so bio-chemical values are used instead. TC is more variable than LDL-C, but even if LDL-C is used, there is an overlap between affected and unaffected children. Those with LDL-C <3.0 mmol/L have almost certainly not inherited the gene, whereas those >3.7 mmol/L proba-bly have. In between there is a zone of uncertainty (Nicholls *et al.*, 2008). In families with a history of premature vascular disease the children should be tested at about 4 yrs old, pre-school, as this gives an opportunity to teach good eating habits.

There is evidence of carotid artery disease in children with HeFH by the age of 11 yrs, manifest as altered intima–media thickness (Wiegman *et al.*, 2004) and endothelial dysfunction (Sorensen *et al.*, 1994), which is reversible (De Jongh *et al.*, 2002). In families with a strong history of premature vascular disease, treatment should begin earlier. Pravastatin is licensed for use from 8 yrs and atorvastatin from 10 yrs onwards (Arambepola *et al.*, 2007). In families with a more benign vascular history, the decision to treat may be deferred until teenage years. However, a recent report from the American Pediatric Association recommends treatment from the age of 10 if the LDL-C is >4.9 despite diet (Daniels and Greer, 2008).

7.6 **Women with FH**

In general, women are less prone than men to develop CHD, at least until the menopause. An exception occurs in FH, when CHD may be manifest at a younger age. Women should therefore be treated in the same way as men. Low oestrogen contraceptive pills, or progesterone-only pills, are acceptable, and so is low-dose oestrogen replacement therapy for menopausal symptoms.

Although there is no direct evidence of teratogenicity, drugs should be avoided in pregnancy, except resins. Statins in particular should be discontinued before planned pregnancy. Lipid levels rise during pregnancy but the hormonal status makes CHD unlikely. Statins transfer into breast milk and should also be avoided during breastfeeding. Otherwise, treatment can be recommenced after delivery. Mothers should be advised to test their children for FH at a pre-school age as there is a one in two chance of inheritance.

7.7 **HoFH**

HoFH is rare in the UK as the odds against it occurring by chance are less than one in a million. Most cases arise in areas where HeFH is more prevalent, or where consanguineous marriages are permitted (Kachadurian, 1964). If two affected individuals mate, then one in four of their children will have HoFH, two HeFH, and one normal. True HoFH occurs when the parents have the same gene defect, as would occur if they came from the same family, whereas the chance meeting of two HeFH patients with different gene defects may produce a 'compound heterozygote'.

In the absence of functioning LDL receptors, cholesterol levels rise to >20 mmol/L, and there are widespread TX, planar, and tuberous xanthomata even in childhood. Untreated, death occurs in teenage years from extensive atherosclerosis. Clearly genetic counselling is advised to avoid such events if at all possible.

The treatment of HoFH is difficult as statins are relatively ineffective. Other drugs such as resins or ezetimibe may help, but many patients require LDL apheresis or plasma exchange in addition (Thompson *et al.*, 1985). Both portacaval shunt and liver transplantation have also been used (Bilheimer et al., 1984). Gene replacement therapy has been attempted in HoFH (Grossman et al., 1994). Liver cells taken from the patient were transfected with adenovirus particles containing the DNA for LDL-R and were re-injected into the portal system. A limited reduction in LDL-C resulted. There will almost certainly be further developments in this area, especially for the genetically determined dyslipidaemias.

7.8 Treatment of HeFH

Patients with FH should be referred to the local Lipid Clinic for treatment and family tracing. Statins are the mainstay of treatment, usually the more powerful atorvastatin or rosuvastatin (see Chapter 9). Even then the maximum doses are unlikely to normalize TC or LDL-C levels, and in turn are associated with more side effects. A submaximal dose is often therefore combined with other treatment such as ezetimibe or a fibrate. Occasionally patients need all three to achieve target, especially if they have known vascular disease. Other agents which have occasional use are nicotinic acid or resins.

References

Abifadel M, Varret M, Rabès J-P et al. (2003). Mutations in PCSK9 cause autosomal dominant hypercholesterolemia. Nat. Genet., 34, 154–6.

Arambepola C, Farmer AJ, Perera R, and Neil HAW (2007). Statin treatment for children and adolescents with heterozygous familial hypercholesterolaemia: a systematic review and meta-analysis. Atherosclerosis, 195, 339–47.

Betteridge DJ, Broome K, Durrington PN et al. (1991). Risk of fatal coronary artery disease in familial hypercholesterolaemia. Scientific Steering Committee on behalf of the Simon Broome Register Group. Br. Med. J., 303, 893–6.

Bilheimer DW, Goldstein JW, Grundy S, Starzl TE, and Brown MS (1984). Liver transplantation to provide low-density lipoprotein receptors and lower plasma cholesterol in a child with homozygous familial hypercholesterolemia. N. Engl. J. Med., 311, 1658–62.

Burns FS (1920) A contribution to the study of the etiology of xanthoma multiplex. Arch. Dermatol. Syphilol., 2, 415–29.

Damgaard D, Larsen ML, Nissen PH et al. (2005). The relationship of molecular genetic to clinical diagnosis of familial hypercholesterolaemia in a Danish population. Atherosclerosis, 180, 155–60.

Daniels SR and Greer FR (2008). Lipid screening and cardiovascular health in childhood. Pediatrics, 122: 198–208.

De Jongh S, Lilien MR, Op't Roodt et al. (2002). Early statin therapy restores endothelial function in children with familial hypercholesterolaemia. J. Am. Coll. Cardiol., 40, 2117–21.

Defesche JC (2000). Familial hypercholesterolaemia. In Betteridge DJ, ed. *Lipids and vascular disease: current issues*, pp. 65–76. Martin Dunitz, London.

DeMott K, Nhehera L, Humphries SE *et al*. (2008). *Clinical guidelines and evidence review for familial hypercholesterolaemia: the identification and management of adults and children with familial hypercholesterolaemia*. National Collaborating Centre for Primary Care and Royal College of General Practitioners, London. www.nice.org.uk.

Department of Health (2003). *Our inheritance, our future*. www.dh.gov.uk/en/Publicationsandstatistics.

Garcia CK, Wilund K, Arca M *et al*. (2001). Autosomal recessive hypercholesterolemia caused by mutations in a putative LDL receptor adaptor protein. *Science*, **292**, 1394–8.

Goldstein JL and Brown MS (1975). Familial hypercholesterolemia: a genetic regulatory defect in cholesterol metabolism. *Am. J. Med*., **58**, 147–50.

Graham CA, McIlhatton BP, Kirk CW *et al*. (2005). Genetic screening protocol for familial hypercholesterolaemia which includes splicing defects gives an improved mutation detection rate. *Atherosclerosis*, **182**, 331–40.

Grossman M, Raper SE, Kozarsky K *et al*. (1994). Successful *ex vivo* gene therapy directed to liver in a patient with familial hypercholesterolemia. *Nat. Genet*., **6**, 335–41.

Kachadurian AK (1964). The inheritance of essential familial hypercholesterolemia. *Am. J. Med*., **37**, 402–7.

Kotze MJ, Davis HJ, Bissbort S, *et al*. (1993). Intrafamilial variability in the clinical expression of familial hypercholesterolemia: importance of risk factor determination for genetic counselling. *Clin. Genet*., **43**: 295–9.

Mohrschladt MF, Westendorp RGJ, Gevers Leuven JA, and Smelt AHM (2004). Cardiovascular disease and mortality in statin-treated patients with familial hypercholesterolaemia. *Atherosclerosis*, **172**, 329–35.

National Institute for Health and Clinical Excellence (NICE) (2008). *Clinical guidelines and evidence review for familial hypercholesterolaemia: the identification and management of adults and children with familial hypercholesterolaemia*. www.nice.org.uk/CG71.

Neil HAW, Hawkins MM, Durrington PN, Betteridge DJ, Capps NE, and Humphries SE (2005). Non-coronary heart disease mortality and risk of fatal cancer in patients with treated heterozygous familial hypercholesterolaemia: a prospective registry study. *Atherosclerosis*, **179**, 293–7.

Neil HAW, Seagroatt V, Betteridge DJ *et al*. (2004). Established and emerging coronary risk factors in patients with heterozygous familial hypercholesterolaemia. *Heart*, **90**, 1431–7.

Nicholls DP (2006). Familial hypercholesterolaemia in children. *Br. J. Cardiol*., **13**, 191–4.

Nicholls DP, Cather M, Byrne C, Graham CA, and Young IS (2008). Diagnosis of heterozygous familial hypercholesterolaemia in children. *Int. J. Clin. Pract*., **62**, 990–4.

Scientific Steering Committee on behalf of the Simon Broome Register Group (1999). Mortality in treated heterozygous familial hypercholesterolaemia: implications for clinical management. *Atherosclerosis*, **142**, 105–12.

Sijbrands EJG, Westendorp RGJ, Defesche JC, de Meier PHEM, Smelt AHM and Kastelein JJP (2001). Mortality over two centuries in large pedigree with familial hypercholesterolaemia: family tree mortality study. *Br. Med. J.*, **322**: 1019–23.

Slack J (1969). Risk of ischaemic heart disease in familial hyperlipoproteinaemic states. *Lancet*, **ii**: 1380–2.

Sorensen KE, Celemajer DS, Georgakopoulos D, Hatcher G, Betteridge DJ, and Deanfield JE (1994). Impairment of endothelium-dependent dilation is an early event in children with familial hypercholesterolemia and is related to the Lipoprotein (a) level. *J. Clin. Invest.*, **93**, 50–5.

Thompson GR, Miller JP, and Breslow JL (1985). Improved survival of patients with homozygous familial hypercholesterolaemia treated with plasma exchange. *Br. Med. J.*, **295**, 1671–3.

Tosi I, Toledo-Leiva P, Neuwirth C, Naoumova RP, and Soutar AK (2007). Genetic defects causing familial hypercholesterolaemia: identification of deletions and duplications in the LDL-receptor gene and summary of all mutations found in patients attending the Hammersmith Hospital Lipid Clinic. *Atherosclerosis*, **194**, 102–11.

Tybjaerg-Hansen A and Humphries SE (1992). Familial defective apolipoprotein B-100: a single mutation that causes hypercholesterolaemia and premature coronary artery disease. *Atherosclerosis*, **96**, 91–107.

Wiegman A, de Groot E, Hutten BA *et al.* (2004). Arterial intima–media thickness in childhood. A study in familial hypercholesterolaemia heterozygotes and their siblings. *Lancet*, **363**, 369–70.

Wierzbicki AS, Humphries SE, and Minhas R (2008). Familial hypercholesterolaemia: summary of NICE guidance. *Br. Med. J.*, **337**, 509–10.

Chapter 8

Hypertriglyceridaemia

Key points

- Triglyceride (TG) levels should be measured fasting.
- Raised TG levels are often secondary to other causes.
- Raised TG levels are atherogenic, especially when combined with high low-density lipoprotein cholesterol (LDL-C) or low high-density lipoprotein cholesterol (HDL-C).
- Very high TG levels (>20 mmol/L) may cause acute pancreatitis.
- The drug treatment of first choice is a fibrate.

8.1 Introduction

By themselves, raised TG levels are only weakly atherogenic (Criqui *et al.*, 1993) but the risk is increased if LDL-C levels are high or HDL-C levels are low. Raised TG levels are often secondary to other causes (see Table 8.1). Clinically the main problem is the potential for developing pancreatitis, but TG levels have to be very high (usually >20 mmol/L). Measuring the area under the postprandial alimentary lipaemia curve, or measuring the TG-rich lipoproteins (TRL, see Chapter 2), may be a more accurate way of assessing TGs rather than a single fasting level.

Table 8.1 Causes of secondary dyslipidaemia

- Hypothyroidism
- Nephrotic syndrome, chronic renal disease
- Diabetes
- Alcohol
- Obesity
- Pregnancy
- Chronic liver disease
- Drugs—isotretinoin, antiretroviral drugs
- Minor changes with β-blockers, diuretics, and oestrogens

8.2 **Mixed hyperlipidaemia**

In this condition (Frederickson type IIb), both LDL-C and TG are elevated. It is now the commonest single reason for referral to a Lipid Clinic. Many cases are secondary to a list of known causes (see Table 8.1) but in some no cause can be identified. Some clearly run in families (see below), but there remains no clear genetic basis for the disorder. There is debate as to whether the lipid abnormality is independently atherogenic, but at least in the case of diabetes and of renal disease, this would seem to be the case.

There are many causes of this very common pattern of dyslipidaemia. Some are self-evident, such as obesity, but others need to be excluded by a careful history (alcohol abuse) or by specific testing, such as diabetes or nephrotic syndrome. Hypothyroidism may not be clinically evident. For many years, before the advent of hormonal tests, total cholesterol (TC) was used as a marker of thyroid status and of response to treatment. More recently, drugs such as isotretinoin in the treatment of acne, and antiretroviral agents used in human immunodeficiency virus (HIV)/acquired immunodeficiency syndrome (AIDS), have been identified as causes of mixed hyperlipidaemia. In some patients, no underlying cause can be found. The LDL-C component of the disorder is atherogenic, but in addition patients with fasting TG levels >20 mmol/L are at risk from pancreatitis (see above).

Clearly the primary treatment of mixed hyperlipidaemia is identification of the underlying cause, if possible. Otherwise, the main treatment is with a fibrate, combined with a statin or nicotinic acid if needed. Some statins such as atorvastatin and rosuvastatin reduce TG as well as TC (see Chapter 9).

8.3 **Familial combined hyperlipidaemia**

FCH is one of the commonest dyslipidaemias, and yet its genetic and biochemical background remains obscure. There is no doubt that mixed hyperlipidaemia may cluster in families and sometimes display an autosomal dominant pattern of inheritance, but so far no single gene cause has been identified, which is in marked contrast to heterozygous familial hypercholesterolaemia (HeFH) (Wierzbicki *et al.*, 2008). Abnormalities in the *Apo A5* gene have been identified (Wright *et al.*, 2006), but much research remains to be done. In the meantime, FCH may be very atherogenic and requires aggressive treatment.

8.4 **Remnant hyperlipidaemia**

This condition has a characteristic biochemical and clinical profile. There is accumulation of intermediate density lipoprotein (IDL), and it is classified as Frederickson type III. It only occurs in apo E_2/E_2 phenotype (see below) and is atherogenic in peripheral as well as coronary vessels. There is marked variability in lipid levels within the individual, especially with body weight.

This unique pattern of dyslipidaemia is due to the inability of apolipoprotein E (apo E) to initiate IDL catabolism, and so IDL accumulates in the blood. IDL is readily identified in the ultracentrifuge (hence the Frederickson classification) and also on electrophoresis, where it appears as a broad pre-β band. Apo E has four phenotypes (and corresponding genotypes), E_{1-4}, but apo E_1 is rare. Most of the population therefore have varying combinations—E_2/E_2, E_2/E_3, E_2/E_4, E_3/E_3, E_3/E_4, or E_4/E_4. Almost all patients with remnant hyperlipidaemia have the phenotype E_2/E_2, which occurs in <2% of the population, but by no means all of the subjects with this phenotype have dyslipidaemia. It would seem that a critical set of circumstances has to occur before dyslipidaemia develops.

The E_4 allele is also associated with premature coronary disease (Schmitz et al., 2007), but the phenotype E_4/E_4 has been associated with the development of premature Alzheimer's disease (Farrer et al., 1997), so the laboratory report is usually 'Apo-E phenotype/genotype is compatible/not compatible with remnant hyperlipidaemia'.

Typically remnant hyperlipidaemia presents with a severe mixed pattern, and more sophisticated tests such as ultracentrifugation and/or apo E phenotyping or genotyping are needed to reveal the underlying abnormality. It may also present with xanthomata in the palmar creases, a unique feature of this disorder (Figure 8.1), or tuberoeruptive xanthomata, especially on the elbows (Figure 8.2). The lipid abnormality may be very variable, ranging from virtually normal to very high levels (TC >10 mmol/L + TG >20 mmol/L) in the same individual, often depending on body weight. It is very atherogenic, especially in peripheral rather than coronary arteries. It can occur along with other lipid problems—patients with HeFH may also have the apo E_2/E_2 phenotype.

Remnant dyslipidaemia responds well to weight reduction and fibrates, and additional medication is rarely needed.

8.5 **Low HDL and raised TG**

The combination of a raised fasting TG and a low HDL-C (<1 mmol/L, raised TC:HDL-C ratio) is also atherogenic (see Chapters 2 and 4). This was highlighted in the PROCAM studies from Germany (Assmann and Schulte, 1992). Although the profile occurred in only 3.7% of the >20,000 patients studied, it was associated with a quarter of the coronary events.

This profile is common in diabetic dyslipidaemia, and responds well to nicotinic acid (see Chapter 9).

Figure 8.1 Palmar crease xanthomata in remnant (type III) dyslipidaemia (see also Colour plate 3)

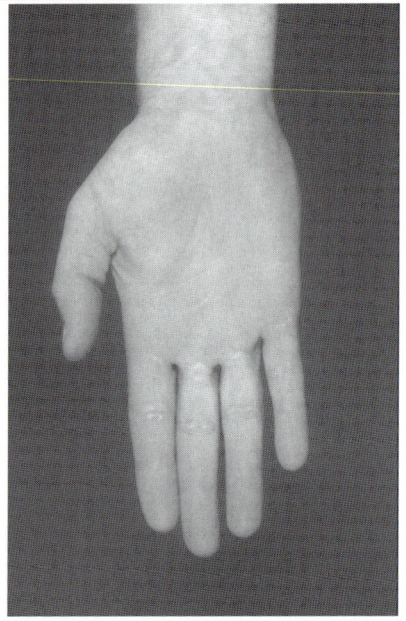

Figure 8.2 Tuboeruptive xanthomata on the elbow of a patient with remnant (type III) hyperlipidaemia (see also Colour plate 4)

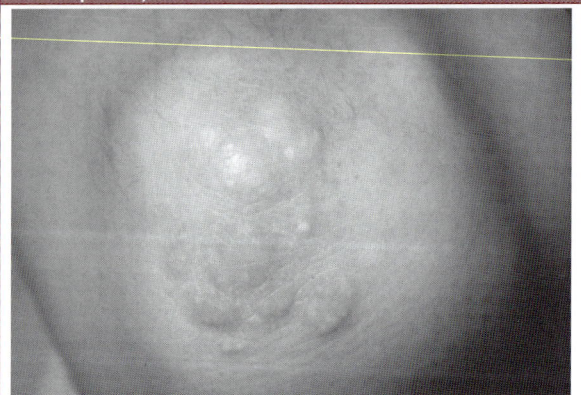

8.6 **Rare lipid disorders**

In addition, there are two much less common disorders characterized by raised TG levels. In childhood, type I hyperlipidaemia is due to the inability to metabolize chylomicrons (chylos), which normally increase after food, due to deficiency of lipoprotein lipase or its co-factor apo C-II. On inspection of the blood, the plasma (or serum) is clear but there is a dense upper layer due to the chylomicrons. Clinically, it presents with recurrent abdominal pains due to pancreatitis, hepato-splenomegaly, and eruptive xanthomata, especially over the buttocks. The retina may appear pale (lipaemia retinalis). The disorder is not atherogenic. Treatment is dietary, and then fibrates with medium-chain triglycerides, although these are unpalatable.

Type V hyperlipidaemia occurs in adults. It is similar to type I hyperlipidaemia (see above) but very low density lipoprotein (VLDL) increased too, giving a turbid serum with a creamy top layer. It is often secondary, especially to alcohol. The main problem remains pancreatitis. It occasionally occurs during pregnancy, which may limit the treatment options. Normally, treatment is with fibrates, fish oils, and occasionally dietary supplementation.

Other clinical syndromes are well recognized, but are rare (Table 8.2). Not all are atherogenic, and indeed some may be protective. For a fuller discussion of these uncommon disorders, see Durrington, 2007.

Table 8.2 Rare lipid disorders

- Atherogenic
  - Apolipoprotein AI–CII deficiency
  - lecithin cholesterol acyltransferase (LCAT) deficiency
  - Hyperapobetalipoproteinaemia (apo B)
- Non-atherogenic
  - Tangier disease
  - Fish-eye disease
- Possibly protective against atherosclerosis
  - A- or hypobetalipoproteinaemia
  - Hyperalphaproteinaemia

References

Assmann G and Schulte H (1992). Relation of high-density lipoprotein cholesterol and triglycerides to incidence of atherosclerotic coronary artery disease (the PROCAM experience). *Am. J. Cardiol.*, **70**, 733–7.

Criqui MH, Heiss G, Cohn, R *et al.* (1993). Plasma triglyceride level and mortality from coronary artery disease. *N. Engl. J. Med.*, **328**, 1220–5.

Durrington PN (2007). *Hyperlipidaemia: diagnosis and management*, 3rd edition. Hodder Arnold, London.

Farrer LA, Cupples A, Haines JL *et al.* (1997). Effects, of age, sex, and ethnicity on the association between apolipoprotein E genotype and Alzheimer's disease. *J. Am. Med. Assoc.*, **278**, 1349–56.

Schmitz F, Mevissen V, Krantz C *et al.* (2007). Robust association of the APOE ε4 allele with premature myocardial infarction especially in patients without hypercholesterolaemia: the Aachen study. *Eur. J. Clin. Invest.*, **37**, 106–8.

Wierzbicki AS, Graham CA, Young IS, and Nicholls DP (2008). Familial combined hyperlipidaemia: under-defined and under-diagnosed? *Curr. Vasc. Pharmacol.*, **6**, 13–22.

Wright WT, Young IS, Nicholls DP, Patterson C, Lyttle K, and Graham CA (2006). SNPs at the *APOA5* gene account for the strong association with hypertriglyceridaemia at the APOA5/A4/C3/A1 locus on chromosome 11q23 in the Northern Irish population. *Atherosclerosis*, **185**, 353–60.

Chapter 9

Treatments available

Key points

- For raised total cholesterol (TC) levels, start with simvastatin.
- If this is not sufficient, change to atorvastatin or rosuvastatin, or add ezetimibe.
- For raised triglyceride (TG) or mixed lipid profiles, start with a fibrate. Add low dose statin later if need be.
- For remnant (type III) hyperlipidaemia, use a fibrate.
- For very high TG levels, use a fibrate and fish oil.
- If high-density lipoprotein (HDL) falls, try nicotinic acid.

9.1 Lifestyle advice

All patients should be offered lifestyle advice as appropriate for the individual, with a view to improving lipids and reducing cardio-vascular risk. This involves healthy eating (see below), regular aerobic exercise, and the avoidance of smoking and excessive alcohol consumption. Cigarette smoking has been identified as a key factor contributing to the morbidity of familial hypercholesterolaemia (FH) (see Chapter 7). There is a range of nicotine patches and tablets that can alleviate withdrawal symptoms, but none are effective without will-power as well. Even if patients cannot stop smoking completely, there is benefit from a reduction in the number smoked each day, and this can materially reduce the cardiovascular risk.

Attention should also be paid to good blood pressure control, the avoidance of obesity (especially in hypertriglyceridaemia), and the detection of glucose intolerance. In patients with overt diabetes, good glycaemic control is essential to achieving a satisfactory lipid profile.

9.2 Dietary intervention

In the UK the percentage of daily calories derived from fat is currently about 37% for men, and slightly less for women (The National Diet and Nutrition Survey, 2002). Whilst this has changed over the past 20 yrs from over 40%, a further reduction in this level would almost

Table 9.1 Sources of dietary fat

Saturated: butter, cheese, lard, suet, ghee, coconut oil, palm oil.

Polyunsaturated: cornflower, soya and sunflower oil, some margarines, fish oil (herring, kippers, mackerel, pilchards, sardines, salmon, trout, and fresh tuna).

Monounsaturated: olive, walnut and rapeseed oils, avocado, some margarines.

Cholesterol: liver, kidneys, egg yolks, sea foods such as prawns.

certainly reduce population cholesterol levels and consequently coronary heart disease (CHD), but is politically difficult. For the individual, to reduce fat intake to 30% is a reasonable target, with a balance of 10% saturated fats, 10% polyunsaturated fats, including fish oils, and 10% monounsaturated fats (see Table 9.1). An increase in fruit, vegetables and fibre, and a reduction in salt intake, is helpful. In addition, patients should be encouraged to eat oily fish at least once a week (see below).

The emphasis is on 'sensible eating'. Extreme low fat diets are unpleasant and have no place except possibly in the treatment of type I or V dyslipidaemia (see Chapter 8). Supplementation with medium-chain TGs is also unpleasant as they taste foul. It is important that the absorption of fat-soluble vitamins (A, D, K) is not impaired. Weight reduction is often an important component, especially in hypertriglyceridaemias. Alcohol in moderation is not a problem and may even help to reduce low-density lipoprotein cholesterol (LDL-C) although this does not seem to be a property of red wine alone.

It should be noted that the achievable reduction in TC is about 15%, which is rarely sufficient on its own in conditions such as heterozygous familial hypercholesterolaemia (HeFH), but forms a useful background to drug treatment. If the initial TC is >6 mmol/L, it is unlikely that diet alone will suffice.

Certain foods do seem to have a beneficial effect, such as types of margarine spread, and odourless garlic.

9.3 **Statins**

Statins were originally derived from fungi as antibiotics, as they interfere with cell wall synthesis in bacteria (Chapter 1). In man, they act by antagonizing intrahepatic β-hydroxy-β-methylglutaryl-coenzyme A reductase (HMG-CoA) reductase, a rate-limiting step in cholesterol synthesis, leading to a reflex increase in LDL receptor (LDL-R) numbers. They differ pharmacologically in their fat solubility and excretion patterns. This does not seem to be important in clinical use, but may affect their liability to produce muscle damage (see Table 9.2). Simvastatin, atorvastatin, and lovastatin are metabolized in the liver by the cytochrome P-450 (CYP) 3A4 pathway, and fluvastatin and rosuvastatin by the CYP 2C9 or 2C19 isoenzymes. There is therefore the potential for interaction with other drugs (such as warfarin) that are metabolized through the same pathway, with either increased circulating levels of the statin or diminished levels of the interacting drug. Pravastatin is also metabolized in the liver but by sulphation and conjugation, so drug interactions are less likely to occur (Muscari et al., 2002). In practice, significant drug interactions are uncommon (see Table 9.3).

In the UK, simvastatin is now 'off patent' and is available generically and 'over the counter'. Cerivastatin was the most potent statin on a molar basis, with doses in the microgram range, but was much more likely to cause myositis than the others and has been withdrawn (Bermingham et al., 2000). Lovastatin is marketed in the USA but not in the UK.

Statins reduce LDL-C with a small increase in HDL cholesterol (HDL-C). There is impressive evidence of efficacy in terms of reduction of cardiovascular events and overall mortality, both in primary and secondary prevention (Cheung et al., 2004; Chapter 12). The newer statins (atorvastatin and rosuvastatin) are more powerful than the older ones (Law et al., 2003; Chapter 12) and hence are of value when large cholesterol reductions are required, as in the treatment of HeFH. They may also help to reduce TG levels as well. The degree of reduction of LDL-C varies from about 25% with simvastatin 10 mg to nearly 60% with atorvastatin 80 mg. Each reduction of LDL-C by 1 mmol/L is associated with a reduction in CVS events by about 20%, but the numbers needed to treat to avoid one such event are greater in primary than in secondary prevention (40 vs 21; Cholesterol Treatment Trialists Collaborators report (CTT Collaborators),

Table 9.2 Liability of statins to produce muscle damage

Cerivastatin +++
Rosuvastatin ++
Atorvastatin, pravastatin, simvastatin +
Fluvastatin −

Table 9.3 Statin drug interactions

- Lipid lowering—fibrates (especially gemfibrozil), nicotinic acid, other statins (!)
- Azol antifungals
- Macrolide antibiotics (quinolones)
- Antivirals
- Ciclosporin, tacrolimus
- Amiodarone, verapamil, possibly diltiazem
- Oestrogen (weak)
- Warfarin? (weak)

2005). In another analysis, a reduction of LDL-C of 1.8 mmol/L resulted in a 60% fall in CHD rates, but a less impressive 17% fall in strokes (Law et al., 2003). In keeping with the philosophy that the lower the LDL-C levels the better (see Chapter 2) there has been recent interest in intensive treatment schedules (see Chapter 12), but it is possible that most of the benefit of such regimes occurs in acute coronary syndromes (ACS) rather than stable chronic CHD (Afilalo et al., 2007).

Lovastatin, simvastatin, and pravastatin have been in use for over 20 yrs, and over this time there has been no evidence of long-term toxicity (Gotto, 2005; Law and Rudnicka, 2006). The same applies to the newer drugs, atorvastatin (Waters, 2005) or rosuvastatin (Alsheikh-Ali et al., 2005). For a fuller discussion on this topic, see also the guidance on the use of statins in cardiovascular disease prevention (NICE, 2006), the report of the National Lipid Association Task Force in the USA (Jacobson and McKenney, 2006), the CTT Collaborators report (2005), the report from the Clinical Trials Unit in Oxford (Armitage, 2007), and the results of recent trials (Ray et al., 2007). In particular, there is no excess of malignancies, which had been a controversial area in earlier lipid-lowering trials (see Chapter 1) (Bonovas et al., 2007).

It is possible that not all the benefit of statin therapy relates to reduction of LDL-C levels, the so-called 'pleiotropic' effect (Topol, 2004), although this area remains controversial (Robinson et al., 2005). In particular, there may be an effect on inflammation, which is an important part of the atherosclerotic process (Sattar et al., 2003; see Chapter 5). Raised levels of C-reactive protein (CRP), a marker of inflammation, are associated with an increase in all-cause mortality (Currie et al., 2008). Statins reduce CRP levels (Ridker et al., 2005), especially in high dose (Nissen et al., 2005), and this is associated with an improved clinical outcome (Ridker et al., 2008).

Concern has been expressed about proteinuria as evidence of renal damage (Deslypere et al., 1990), but this may reflect a physiological action of statins on protein reabsorption in the renal tubule (Agarwal, 2006). Patients with chronic kidney disease (CKD), especially end-stage renal disease (ESRD), often have dyslipidaemia characterized by highly atherogenic small dense LDL-C particles (Cheung et al., 1993), and they are very prone to cardiovascular complications (Foley and Collins, 2007). Statins reduce cardiovascular events in patients with CKD as they do in the general population (Strippoli et al., 2008), although the position in patients with ESRD is not yet clear (Clase, 2008). Long-term follow-up of patients on statins has not shown an excess of deaths from renal failure (see safety studies earlier).

The side-effect profile of statins is remarkably low and merges into placebo rates in most trials. A moderate (up to 3 × upper limit of normal) increase in the liver enzymes aspartate aminotransferase (AST) and alanine aminotransferase (ALT) often occurs and is reversible if the drug is discontinued. γGT is not affected (see Chapter 10). Statins may reduce gallstone formation. There is no evidence of long-term liver damage (Cash et al., 2008).

The only other consistent finding is of myositis, which can also occur with fibrates and nicotinic acid (see Chapter 11). Minor degrees are not uncommon but frank rhabdomyolysis is rare, occurring in <1 case per 10,000 patients on treatment (Armitage, 2007). Not all statins are equal in this respect (see Table 9.2) and the differences probably relate to the solubility and excretion patterns noted earlier. Myositis is more likely to occur under certain circumstances (Table 9.4).

Statin therapy is well tolerated in the majority of patients, but a significant minority (about 5% to 10%) have problems (Simons et al., 1996; Nair et al, 2008), most commonly with myalgia. In most cases, these can be resolved without recourse to discontinuation. A suggested plan of action is shown in Table 9.5.

Table 9.4 Myositis more likely

- Elderly, frail patients
- Asians
- Renal disease
- Hypothyroid
- High dose
- Other drugs (Table 9.3)
- Genetic predisposition (Chapter 11)

Table 9.5 Statin intolerance

- Is lipid lowering therapy really needed, for example for secondary prevention (see Chapter 6)?
- Is there a temporal relationship between the symptoms and the treatment?
- Did the total creatine kinase (tCK) levels remain normal throughout?
- If treatment is definitely indicated, there is no clear relationship of symptoms to starting and stopping treatment, and there is no objective evidence of myositis, then reassurance may be sufficient.
- If not, try another statin—the difference in the pharmacokinetic profiles means that not all are the same.
- Start with a very low dose, for example rosuvastatin 5 mg and increase slowly—or try once weekly treatment at first.
- Reduce the dose of statin and combine with ezetimibe or a fibrate.
- Coenzyme Q10 supplements may be tried but proof of efficacy is lacking (see Chapter 11).

Table 9.6 Fibrate formulations

Bezafibrate	200 mg tablets three times daily and 400 mg m/r tablets once daily
Ciprofibrate	100 mg tablets daily
Fenofibrate	67 mg capsules 2–4 times a day, 200 mg or 267 mg capsules once daily, 160 mg tablets once daily
Gemfibrozil	300 mg capsules or 600 mg tablets both twice daily

N.B. Once daily doses should be taken with evening meal.

9.4 **Fibrates**

Clofibrate (now withdrawn) was introduced in 1962 and was the first drug specifically designed to lower lipid levels. Bezafibrate, gemfibrozil, ciprofibrate, and fenofibrate followed (Table 9.6). They share a common mode of action, which includes activation of peroxisome proliferator-activated receptors (PPAR), especially PPARα (Chapman, 2006). This leads to reduced hepatic TG synthesis, increased lipoprotein lipase activity and hence VLDL clearance, increased clearance of remnant particles, and increased levels of HDL-C. In addition, small dense LDL-C is converted to a lighter, more buoyant form, which is less atherogenic. This profile of action is potentially beneficial, especially in patients with Type 2 diabetes or the metabolic syndrome (Chapman, 2006).

They are the drugs of choice when TG levels are raised, or in combination with statins in mixed hyperlipidaemias (see Chapter 8). The evidence of benefit is less clear than after statins (Wierzbicki, 2006) although there is a reduction in new vascular events in secondary prevention (Frick et al., 1987; Chapter 12). There is a moderate reduction in LDL-C and HDL-C levels usually increase (UK HDL-C Consensus Group, 2004). Occasionally, HDL-C levels may fall markedly. The reason for this adverse reaction remains unclear but may have a genetic basis. A change to nicotinic acid is then usually indicated (see Section 9.6 later).

Their main problem is dyspepsia, and fibrates may also increase gallstone formation. Caution should be exercised in renal disease or hypothyroidism. They are uniquely effective in the treatment of remnant (type III) hyperlipidaemia (see Chapter 8). Used alone, fibrates rarely cause myositis, but there was an increased rate with the combination of gemfibrozil and statins, especially cerivastatin (Bermingham et al., 2000), which has since been withdrawn.

9.5 **Ezetimibe**

This acts as a specific cholesterol absorption inhibitor in the small bowel, independently of acyl CoA cholesteryl acyl transferase (ACAT). It acts on Niemann-Pick C1-like 1, a critical mediator of cholesterol absorption from the gut (Garcia-Calvo et al., 2005). The effect on TC is equivalent to a strict diet—about 15% reduction. In terms of LDL-C reduction, there is an additive effect to statins and fibrates, but there is recent controversy about whether this is translated into clinical benefit (Brown and Taylor, 2008; Kastelein et al., 2008). There does not appear to be an added risk of myositis when added to a statin (Davidson et al., 2006), but there have been reports of hepatotoxicity (Stolk et al., 2006). Overall, the adverse event profile of ezetimibe is low (Florentin et al., 2008).

The current recommendations are that ezetimibe may be used in addition to a statin when targets have not been met, or when there is statin intolerance (Wierzbicki et al., 2005). Ezetimibe monotherapy may also be used in this situation (NICE, 2007). Ezetimibe may be of value in the treatment of homozygous familial hypercholesterolaemia (HoFH) (see Chapter 7). Single dose = 10 mg daily or as combination with simvastatin (Inegy®; Vytorin™ in the USA).

A recent study has cast doubt on whether the addition of ezetimibe to a statin confers any added benefit in terms of event reduction (Kastelein et al., 2008), but the conclusions are not universally accepted. In addition, a recent study of lipid lowering in patients with aortic stenosis treated with ezetimibe or placebo (Rossebø et al., 2008) did not show any benefit, but did suggest an increase in cancers (of all types). Overall, the risk of developing cancer on ezetimibe treatment does not seem to be significantly increased (Peto et al., 2008), but clearly long-term follow-up is required.

9.6 **Nicotinic acid**

Nicotinic acid is related to nicotinamide, part of the vitamin B group. It has been available in the USA for many years but only recently introduced into the UK as Niaspan®. It acts by a reduction in very low density lipoprotein (VLDL) synthesis. There is good evidence for a long-term reduction in mortality when used as secondary prevention (CPD trials, see Chapter 12). Nicotinic acid produces a moderate reduction in TC, a rise in HDL-C, and a considerable reduction in TG. Lp(a) levels may also be decreased (Chapter 3).

A prominent side effect is cutaneous vasodilation, often starting in the face and spreading. The effect seems to be harmless but can be spectacular. Flushing can almost be regarded as a marker of efficacy. It is mediated by prostaglandins and so is prevented by aspirin. There is

Table 9.7 Dosing schedule for nicotinic acid m/r tablets
• 375 mg at night for a week
• 500 mg at night for a week
• 750 mg at night for a week
• 1 g at night for a month
• Increase up to 2 g daily if need, in 500 mg steps at monthly intervals
• A starter pack with instructions is available

marked inter-individual variability—some patients never flush, others find it persistent and unpleasant. It decreases with time. To minimize this effect, start treatment with a low dose of nicotinic acid and increase gradually over a period of weeks to a maximum dose of 2 g daily (Table 9.7). It is best to take the treatment at bed time, and to take aspirin half an hour beforehand. Newer prostaglandin inhibitors such as laropiprant (MK-0524), which do not have the gastrointestinal side effects of aspirin (Cheng *et al.*, 2006), are used in the combined preparation *Tredaptive*.

Glucose levels increase, but not enough to cause diabetes. In established diabetics, a small adjustment of their hypoglycaemic treatment is usually sufficient. Liver function tests may be disturbed, and myositis may rarely occur.

Nicotinic acid is also available as acipimox 250 mg, but this is less effective, probably due to the lower dose used.

9.7 Resins

Anion-exchange resins bind bile salts in the gut producing negative cholesterol balance. They are available as colestyramine or colestipol, and more recently in tablet form as colesevelam. Their efficacy has been recognized for many years (see CDP and LRC-CPPT trials, Chapter 12), but despite effort to make them more palatable, patients find it difficult to take the amount needed to produce a significant reduction in TC (typically 6–8 sachets a day). Their texture is unpleasant but can be disguised by leaving in fruit juice overnight, or taking them along with breakfast cereals. Colesevelam does not appear to have these problems, and can be combined with other treatment such as ezetimibe when statins cannot be used (Zema, 2005).

Resins are now outmoded as single agents but may have an occasional place in low dose as part of a combination strategy, for example in HeFH. They are still used in gastroenterological problems such as itching from obstructive jaundice. They may cause malabsorption of vitamins and drugs and interact with warfarin, and so their administration needs to be carefully timed. In addition, they are expensive.

9.8 **Fish oils**

These reduce overall TG levels and alter TG composition by substituting marine oils (ω-3 TG). They may alter platelet function. There is evidence of benefit after myocardial infarction (GISSI-Prevenzione Investigators, 1999) and also a reduction in restenosis rate after coronary artery angioplasty (Dehmer *et al.*, 1988). A recent study from Japan has shown that the addition of eicosapentaenoic acid to low dose statin therapy significantly reduced new coronary events, especially when used as secondary prevention (Yokoyama *et al.*, 2007).

Fish oil is available as ω-3 marine TG (*Maxepa*, 5 mL [5 capsules] twice daily) or ω-3-acid ethyl esters (*Omacor*, 2–4 capsules daily). Both preparations are relatively expensive because of the careful preparation needed to avoid toxic oxidation. Cod liver oil may also be effective, and patients should be encouraged to eat oily fish (mackerel, kippers, salmon, trout, pilchards, or fresh rather then tinned tuna) at least once a week as part of their diet (see Table 9.1).

9.9 **Invasive treatments**

Plasma exchange is relatively simple but non-selective. It is of occasional use when drug treatment has failed or cannot be tolerated, mainly in HoFH and severe hypertriglyceridaemia with recurrent pancreatitis (Thompson *et al.*, 1985). In that context it is very effective but needs frequent venous access, for example every 2 weeks, otherwise levels rise again. LDL apheresis is similar but uses filter canisters to selectively remove LDL-C alone. Continued use is very expensive. There are similar problems with Heparin Extracorporeal LDL Precipitation (*HELP*), in which blood is dialysed against a low pH buffer, and LDL-C (and fibrinogen) precipitated. As a result of these limitations, such treatment is now confined to specialized centres.

Partial ileal bypass is very effective at reducing LDL-C, as demonstrated in the POSCH study (Buchwald *et al.*, 1990). It was used in refractory HeFH before statins became available and acts by interrupting bile salt cycling. Post-operative diarrhoea is a major problem, with weight loss, and vitamin B12 needs to be replaced. Such operative interventions are now outmoded.

9.10 **New drugs**

As mentioned in Chapter 4, cholesteryl ester transfer protein (CETP) inhibition could potentially increase HDL-C levels, with a favourable effect on CV risk, especially in patients with raised TG levels as well (Dullaart *et al.*, 2007). The first drug in this class (torcetrapib) was recently reported as being associated with increased aldosterone levels, hypertension, and increased deaths and CV events (Barter *et al.*, 2007). It is possible that other members of the class may not have the same effects, and initial reports are encouraging (Stein *et al.*, 2008).

Lipoprotein-associated phospholipase (Lp-PLA$_2$; see Chapter 5) enzymes modify LDL-C particles by hydrolysis, encouraging uptake by macrophages and the initiation of the atherosclerotic process (see Chapter 5). Darapladib and varespladib are inhibitors of Lp-PLA$_2$ and so are under evaluation as anti-atheroma drugs. Initial safety data are encouraging but there are no outcome data available yet.

9.11 **Management—general points**

Be sure you can justify treatment, either as secondary prevention, or primary if the risk is high enough. There is no reason to treat individuals with moderately raised levels who are at low risk (see Chapter 6). Start by offering general lifestyle advice as appropriate and ensuring that the diet is reasonable, but for many patients this means only minor adjustments. In addition, do not treat dyslipidaemia in isolation—attention to the other key risk factors for CHD is essential as part of a holistic approach.

Before starting drugs, discuss the nature and purpose of preventive medication with the patient so that they fully understand the need for treatment. This greatly improves subsequent compliance. Always measure a full lipid profile before treating, including TC, HDL-C, derived LDL-C, and TG. If TG levels are raised, repeat fasting. Always measure liver enzymes (AST, ALT, and gamma-glutamyl transpeptidase (γGT)) and CK before starting treatment—it saves a lot of discussion later. Monitor these tests at 1, 3, and 6 months after starting or changing treatment, and each 6 months thereafter.

9.12 **Raised cholesterol**

The drugs of choice are the statins. Generic simvastatin is by far the least expensive, and has a good trials and safety record, so it is reasonable to start with simvastatin 20 mg daily, increasing to 40 mg if the TC is still raised at 1 month. For patients with initial TC <6 mmol/L, this may suffice. Pravastatin and fluvastatin are also effective in mild to moderate hypercholesterolaemia. Patients with TC >6 mmol/L, such as those with HeFH, should start on a more potent statin such as atorvastatin or rosuvastatin and the dose titrated as required. The highest recommended dose (atorvastatin 80 mg or rosuvastatin 40 mg) is associated with more side effects and hence compliance problems, and so it is probably better to stop at 40 or

Table 9.8 Who to refer to a Lipid Clinic
• Suspected FH or familial combined hyperlipidaemia (FCH)
• Severe hypertriglyceridaemia
• Dyslipidaemia of pregnancy
• Failure to meet targets in secondary prevention

20 mg, respectively, and consider adding in other drugs (combination therapy). The concept of combination therapy is well accepted in the treatment of hypertension.

Few patients with polygenic hypercholesterolaemia fail to respond to these doses, and so it is an appropriate time to reassess the possibility of secondary hyperlipidaemia, whether compliance is satisfactory, or whether the patient has HeFH. Consider whether the patient should be referred to a Lipid Clinic for specialist advice.

The next step is to add in either ezetimibe 10 mg daily or a fibrate. The addition of the latter gives an additive risk of myositis, although the risk is still small. If levels are still not at target, add the other (ezetimibe or fibrate) as well—triple therapy. Still in reserve are small doses of resins (say 2 sachets a day), colesevelam, or nicotinic acid.

9.13 **Mixed hyperlipidaemias**

Be careful to identify and treat the many factors which may cause secondary dyslipidaemia, in particular obesity and alcohol (see Table 8.1). Rule out hypothyroidism and renal disease by biochemical testing. Start with a fibrate. If levels still too high, add in low dose statin, such as atorvastatin 10 mg. If levels are still high, refer to Lipid Clinic for further advice. The next step would probably be nicotinic acid, especially if HDL-C levels are low.

9.14 **Raised TG**

Rule out secondary causes as earlier, and remember that very high levels (>20 mmol/L) are dangerous and demand rapid reduction. Start with a fibrate, and if levels are still raised, add fish oil. If levels still raised, try nicotinic acid. If levels are still high, refer to the Lipid Clinic (Table 9.8).

References

Afilalo J, Majdan AA, and Eisenberg MJ (2007). Intensive statin therapy in acute coronary syndromes and stable coronary artery disease: a comparative meta-analysis of randomised controlled clinical trials. *Heart*, **93**, 914–21.

Agarwal R (2006). Effects of statins on renal function. *Am. J. Cardiol.*, **97**, 748–55.

Alsheikh-Ali AA, Ambrose MS, Kuvin JT, and Karas RH (2005). The safety of rosuvastatin as used in common clinical practice. A postmarketing analysis. *Circulation*, **111**, 3051–7.

Armitage J (2007). The safety of statins in clinical practice. *Lancet*, **370**, 1781–90.

Barter PJ, Caulfield M, Eriksson M *et al.* (ILLUMINATE Investigators) (2007). Effects of torcetrapib in patients at high risk for coronary events. *New Engl. J. Med.*, **357**, 2109–22.

Bermingham RP, Whitsitt TB, Smart ML *et al.* (2000). Rhabdomyolysis in a patient receiving the combination of cerivastatin and gemfibrozil. *Am. J. Health-System Pharm.*, **57**, 461–4.

Bonovas S, Filioussi K, Tsantes A, and Sitaras NM (2007). Use of statins and haematological malignancies: a meta-analysis of six randomized clinical trials and eight observational studies. *Br. J. Clin. Pharmacol.*, **64**, 255–62.

Brown GB and Taylor AJ (2008). Does ENHANCE diminish confidence in lowering LDL or in ezetimibe? *N. Engl. J. Med.*, **358**, 1504–7.

Buchwald H, Varco RL, Matts JP *et al.* (1990). Effect of partial ileal bypass surgery on mortality and morbidity from coronary heart disease in patients with hypercholesterolemia. Report of the Program on the Surgical Control of the Hyperlipidemias (POSCH). *N. Engl. J. Med.*, **323**, 946–55.

Cash J, Callender ME, McDougall NI, Young IS, and Nicholls DP (2008). Statin therapy and chronic liver disease. *Int. J. Clin. Pract.*, **62**: 1831–5.

Chapman MJ (2006). Fibrates: therapeutic review. *Br. J. Diabetes Vasc. Dis.*, **6**: 11–20.

Cheng K, Wu TJ, Wu KK *et al.* (2006). Antagonism of the prostaglandin D2 receptor 1 suppresses nicotinic acid-induced vasodilation in mice and humans. *Proc. Natl. Acad. Sci. USA*, **106**, 6682–7.

Cheung AK, Wu LL, Kablitz C, and Leypoldt JK (1993). Atherogenic lipids and lipoproteins in hemodialysis patients. *Am. J. Kidney Dis.*, **22**, 271–6.

Cheung BMY, Lauder IJ, Lau C-P, and Kumana CR (2004). Meta-analysis of large randomized controlled trials to evaluate the impact of statins on cardiovascular outcomes. *Br. J. Clin. Pharmacol.*, **57**, 640–51.

Cholesterol Treatment Trialists Collaborators (2005). Efficacy and safety of cholesterol-lowering treatment: prospective meta-analysis of data from 90 056 participants in 14 randomised trials of statins. *Lancet*, **366**, 1267–78.

Clase M (2008). Statins for people with kidney disease. *Br. Med. J.*, **336**, 624–5.

Currie CJ, Poole CD, and Conway P (2008). Evaluation of the association between the first observation and the longitudinal change in C-reactive protein, and all-cause mortality. *Heart*, **94**, 457–62.

Davidson MH, Maccubbin D, Stepanavage M, Strony J, and Musliner T (2006). Striated muscle safety of ezetimibe/simvastatin (*Vytorin*). *Am. J. Cardiol.*, **97**, 223–8.

Dehmer GJ, Popma JJ, van den Berg EK et al. (1988). Reduction in the rate of early restenosis after coronary angioplasty by a diet supplemented with n-3 fatty acids. N. Engl. J. Med., **319**, 733–40.

Deslypere JP, Delanghe J, and Vermeulen A (1990). Proteinuria as a complication of simvastatin treatment. Lancet, **336**, 1453.

Dullaart RPF, Dallinga-Thie GM, Wolffenbuttel BHR, and van Tol A (2007). CETP inhibition in cardiovascular risk management: a critical appraisal. Eur. J. Clin. Invest., **37**, 90–8.

Florentin M, Liberopoulos EN, and Elisaf MS (2008). Ezetimibe-associated adverse effects: what the clinician needs to know. Int. J. Clin. Pract., **62**, 88–96.

Foley RN and Collins AJ (2007). End-stage renal disease in the United States: an update form the United States renal data system. J. Am. Soc. Nephrol., **18**, 2644–8.

Garcia-Calvo M, Lisnock J-M, Bull HG et al. (2005). The target of ezetimibe is Niemann-Pick C1-Like 1 (NPC1L1). Proc. Natl. Acad. Sci. USA, **102**, 8132–7.

GISSI-Prevenzione Investigators (1999). Dietary supplementation with n-3 polyunsaturated fatty acids and vitamin E after myocardial infarction: results of the GISSI-Prevenzione trial. Lancet, **354**, 447–55.

Gotto AM (2005). Review of primary and secondary prevention trials with lovastatin, pravastatin, and simvastatin. Am. J. Cardiol., **96**, 34F–38F.

Jacobson TA and McKenney JM (2006). Overview: recommendations of the statin safety task force and benefit:risk considerations with statin therapy. www.medscape.com/viewarticle/548530.

Kastelein JJ, Akdim F, Stroes ES et al. (2008). Simvastatin with or without ezetimibe in familial hypercholesterolemia (ENHANCE). N. Engl. J. Med., **358**, 1431–43.

Law M and Rudnicka AR (2006). Statin safety: a systematic review. Am. J. Cardiol., **97**, 52C–60C.

Law MR, Wald NJ, and Rudnicka AR (2003). Quantifying effect of statins on low density lipoprotein cholesterol, ischaemic heart disease, and stroke: systematic review and meta-analysis. Br. Med. J., **326**, 1423–7.

Muscari A, Puddu GM, and Puddu P (2002). Lipid-lowering drugs: are adverse effects predictable and reversible? Cardiology, **97**, 115–21.

Nair RK, Karadi RL, and Kilpatrick ES (2008). Managing patients with 'statin intolerance': a retrospective study. Br. J. Cardiol., **15**, 158–60.

NICE (National Institute for Health and Clinical Excellence) (2007). Ezetimibe for the treatment of primary (heterozygous familial and non-familial) hypercholesterolaemia. www.nice.org.uk.

NICE (National Institute for Health and Clinical Excellence) (2006). Statins for the prevention of cardiovascular events. www.nice.org.uk.

Nissen SE, Tuzcu EM, Schoenhagen P et al. (2005). Statin therapy, LDL cholesterol, C-reactive protein, and coronary artery disease. N. Engl. J. Med., **352**, 29–38.

Peto R, Emberson J, Landray M, Baigent C, Collins R, Clare R, and Califf R (2008). Analyses of cancer data from three ezetimibe trials. *N. Engl. J. Med.*, **359**, 1357–66.

Ray KK, Cannon CP, and Braunwald E (2007). Recent trials of lipid lowering. *Int. J. Clin. Pract.*, **61**, 1145–59.

Ridker PM, Cannon CP, Morrow D *et al.* (2005). C-reactive protein levels and outcomes after statin therapy. *N. Engl. J. Med.*, **352**, 20–8.

Ridker PM, Danielson E, Francisco AH, *et al.* (2008). Rosuvastatin to prevent vascular events in men and women with elevated C-reactive protein. *N. Engl. J. Med.*, **359**: 2195–2207.

Robinson JG, Smith B, Maheshwari N, and Schrott H (2005). Pleiotropic effect of statins: benefit beyond cholesterol reduction? *J. Am. Coll. Cardiol.*, **46**, 1855–62.

Rossebø AB, Pedersen TR, Borman K *et al.* (2008). Intensive lipid lowering with simvastatin and ezetimibe in aortic stenosis. *N. Engl. J. Med.*, **359**, 1343–56.

Sattar N, McCarey DW, Capell H *et al.* (2003). Explaining how "high-grade" systemic inflammation accelerates vascular risk in rheumatoid arthritis. *Circulation*, **108**, 2957–63.

Simons LA, Levis G, and Simons J (1996). Apparent discontinuation rates in patients prescribed lipid-lowering drugs. *Med. J. Aust.*, **164**, 208–11.

Stein EA, Kallend D, Buckley B, *et al.* (2008). Safety profile of the cholesteryl ester transfer protein inhibitor R1658/JTT-705 in patients with type II hyperlipidemia, or coronary heart disease. *J. Am. Coll. Cardiol.*, **51** (Suppl. A): A333–4.

Stolk MFJ, Becx MCJM, Kuypers KC, and Seldenrijk CA (2006). Severe hepatic side-effects of ezetimibe. *Clin. Gastroenterol. Hepatol.*, **4**, 908–11.

Strippoli GF, Navaneethan SD, Johnson DW *et al.* (2008). Effects of statins in patients with chronic kidney disease: meta-analysis and meta-regression of randomised controlled trials. *Br. Med. J.*, **336**, 645–51.

The National Diet and Nutrition Survey: adults aged 19–64 years (2002). Office for National Statistics, Stationery Office, London.

Thompson GR, Miller JP, and Breslow JL (1985). Improved survival of patients with homozygous familial hypercholesterolaemia treated with plasma exchange. *Br. Med. J.*, **295**, 1671–3.

Topol EJ (2004). Intensive statin therapy—a sea change in cardiovascular disease prevention. *N. Engl. J. Med.*, **350**, 1562–4.

UK HDL-C Consensus Group (2004). Role of fibrates in reducing coronary risk: a UK consensus. *Curr. Med. Res. Opin.*, **20**, 241–7.

Waters DD (2005). Safety of high-dose atorvastatin therapy. *Am. J. Cardiol.*, **97**, 69F–75F.

Wierzbicki AS, Doherty E, Lamb PJ *et al.* (2005). Efficacy of ezetimibe in patients with statin-resistant and statin-intolerant familial hypercholesterolaemia. *Curr. Med. Res. Opin.*, **21**, 333–8.

Wierzbicki AS (2006). FIELDS of dreams, fields of tears: a perspective on the fibrate trials. *Int. J. Clin. Pract.*, **60**: 442–9.

Yokoyama M, Origasa H, Matsuzaki M *et al.* (2007). Effects of eicosapentaenoic acid on major coronary events in hypercholesterolaemic patients (JELIS): a randomised open-label, blinded endpoint analysis. *Lancet*, **369**, 1090–98.

Zema MJ (2005). Colesevelam HCl and ezetimibe combination therapy provides effective lipid-lowering in difficult-to-treat patients with hypercholesterolemia. *Am. J. Therapeut.*, **12**, 306–10.

Chapter 10

Abnormal liver tests

> **Key points**
>
> - Minor elevations of aspartate aminotransferase (AST) and alanine aminotransferase (ALT) occur frequently after statins.
> - Fibrates and nicotinic acid may also disturb liver function tests (LFTs).
> - There is no evidence of long-term liver damage after statin therapy.
> - Raised GGT levels are not due to a statin.
> - Patients with mild or moderate chronic liver disease may also qualify for statin treatment.

10.1 Raised liver enzymes

Statin therapy is frequently associated with elevated levels of AST and ALT (see review by Cash *et al.*, 2008). This appears to be a class effect of statins (Farmer and Torre-Amione, 2000) and may be due to reduced mevalonate levels in the liver secondary to β-hydroxy-β-methylglutaryl-coenzyme A reductase (HMG-CoA) reductase inhibition (Kornbrust *et al.*, 1989). Elevations up to three times the upper limit of normal do not appear to be associated with liver damage, and are not an indication for withdrawing treatment. Levels may stabilize or even normalize with continued use (Chalasani, 2005). From the long-term safety evaluations of statins (see Chapter 9), there are no indications of long-term liver damage or malignancy following continued statin use (see Table 10.1).

> **Table 10.1 Statins and liver tests**
>
> - Liver enzymes (ALT, AST) should be checked before commencing statin treatment, 6–8 weeks later, and annually thereafter.
> - Statins should only be discontinued if they rise to more than three times the upper limit of normal.
> - An isolated rise in γGT or bilirubin is unlikely to be due to statin treatment.
> - Statins may be used safely in stable chronic liver disease, but not in acute or advanced liver disease.

Elevations in transaminases to greater than three times the upper limit of normal are uncommon, occurring in about 2% of patients on statin treatment. The effect does seem to be dose-dependent. In the MIRACL trial of atorvastatin, the rate was 0.2% with 10 mg and 2.3% with 80 mg (Schwarz *et al.*, 2001). Similar effects have been noted with other statins, such as fluvastatin (Serruys *et al.*, 2002). Such elevations may be more common after rosuvastatin (Kasliwal *et al.*, 2007). The abnormalities were usually asymptomatic, occurred shortly after commencing treatment, and normalized after discontinuation. It is recommended that statin treatment is stopped if such elevations are found.

Both nicotinic acid and ezetimibe may also be hepatotoxic on occasion (see Chapter 9).

10.2 **Elevated γGT**

No study has described elevations in gamma-glutamyl transpeptidase (γGT), and an isolated rise in this enzyme is almost certainly not due to statin treatment. The most common cause remains excess alcohol consumption, and this would be supported by the history and the finding of an isolated raised mean corpuscular volume (MCV) on the full blood count. If this is not the cause, an ultrasound scan of the liver would disclose gall stones or fatty changes due to non-alcoholic fatty liver disease (NAFLD) or non-alcoholic steatohepatitis (NASH). It is also worth checking for the presence of anti-mitochondrial antibodies, and to screen for viral hepatitis. On occasion, no cause can be found. An elevated level of γGT is not a contra-indication for statin treatment, nor is it a reason for discontinuation.

10.3 **Liver toxicity**

Severe liver damage is rare after statins, but has been described (Clarke and Mills, 2006). However, the rate of liver failure is similar to that in the general population (Tolman, 2002) and does not appear to be predicted by previous blood tests (McKenney *et al.*, 2006). The liver damage appears to be autoimmune in origin, and is at least partly reversible following withdrawal of the statin (Kasliwal *et al.*, 2007).

10.4 **Use in chronic liver disease**

Patients with mild liver disease, as manifest by elevated bilirubin or enzyme levels, are not at risk from further statin-induced liver damage (Vuppalanchi and Chalasani, 2006). Statins appear to be safe in patients with hepatitis C infection (Khosharadi *et al.*, 2006) or primary biliary cirrhosis (Stojakovic *et al.*, 2007). Patients with NAFLD or NASH may benefit from statin therapy because of their increased risk of cardiovascular disease (Kiyici *et al.*, 2003; Rallidis *et al.*, 2004). As a result of such evidence, the current recommendation of the US National Lipid Association Task Force is that statins are not contra-indicated in patients with chronic liver disease and Child's A cirrhosis (Cohen *et al.*, 2006). Their recommendations are summarized in Table 10.2.

This is of practical importance because many such patients have concurrent cardiovascular disease and so would qualify for statin treatment.

Table 10.2 Statins in patients with liver disease

- Statins may be used in patients with an isolated elevation in γGT or bilirubin, and in those with a normal albumin level and no clinical evidence of liver disease.
- Patients with NAFLD/NASH or genetic liver disease such as haemochromatosis may be treated if the ALT and AST are less than three times the upper limit of normal.
- Use of statins in patients with higher enzyme levels needs careful consideration.
- Use in patients with acute or advanced liver disease remains contra-indicated.

References

Cash J, Callender ME, McDougall NI, Young IS, and Nicholls DP (2008). Statin therapy and chronic liver disease. *Int. J. Clin. Pract.*, **62**: 1831–15.

Chalasani N (2005). Statins and hepatotoxicity: focus on patients with fatty liver. *Hepatology*, **41**, 690–5.

Clarke AT and Mills PR (2006). Atorvastatin associated liver disease. *Dig. Liver Dis.*, **38**, 772–7.

Cohen DE, Anania FA, and Chalasani N (2006). An assessment of statin safety by hepatologists. *Am. J. Cardiol.*, **97**, 77C–81C.

Farmer JA and Torre-Amione G (2000). Comparative tolerability of the HMG-CoA reductase inhibitors. *Drug Saf.*, **23**, 197–213.

Kasliwal R, Wilton LV, Cornelius V, Aurich-Barrera B, and Shakir SA (2007). Safety profile of rosuvastatin: results of a prescription-event study of 11,680 patients. *Drug Saf.*, **30**, 157–70.

Khosharadi S, Hasson NK, and Cheung RC (2006). Incidence of statin hepatotoxicity in patients with hepatitis C. *Clin. Gastroenterol. Hepatol.*, **4**, 902–7.

Kiyici M, Gulte M, Gurel S *et al.* (2003). Ursodeoxycholic acid and atorvastatin in the treatment of non-alcoholic steatohepatitis. *Can. J. Gastroenterol.*, **17**, 713–8.

Kornbrust DJ, MacDonald JS, Peter CP *et al.* (1989). Toxicity of the HMG-coenzyme A reductase inhibitor, lovastatin, to rabbits. *Journal of Pharmacol. Exp. Ther.*, **248**, 498–505.

McKenney JM, Davidson MH, Jacobson TA, and Guyton JR (2006). Final conclusions and recommendations of the National Lipid Association Statin Safety Assessment Task Force. *Am. J. Cardiol.*, **97**, 89C–94C.

Rallidis LS, Drakoulis CK, and Parasi AS (2004). Pravastatin in patients with non-alcoholic steatohepatitis: results of a pilot study. *Atherosclerosis*, **174**, 193–6.

Schwarz GG, Olsson AG, Ezekowitz MD *et al.* (2001). Effects of atorvastatin on early recurrent ischemic events in acute coronary syndromes: the MIRACL study: a randomized controlled trial. *J. Am. Med. Assoc.*, **285**, 1711–8.

Serruys PW, de Feyter P, Macaya C *et al.* (2002). Fluvastatin for prevention of cardiac events following successful first percutaneous coronary intervention: a randomized controlled trial. *J. Am. Med. Assoc.*, **287**, 3215–22.

Stojakovic T, Putz-Bankuti C, Fauler G *et al.* (2007). Atorvastatin in patients with primary biliary cirrhosis and incomplete biochemical response to ursodeoxycholic acid. *Hepatology*, **46**, 776–84.

Tolman KG (2002). The liver and lovastatin. *Am. J. Cardiol.*, **89**, 1374–80.

Vuppalanchi R and Chalasani N (2006). Statins for hyperlipidemia in patients with chronic liver disease: are they safe? *Clin. Gastroenterol. Hepatol.*, **4**, 838–9.

Chapter 11

Muscle pains and CK

Key points

- Myalgia may occur after lipid-lowering treatment, especially statins.
- True myositis is accompanied by a raised creatine kinase (CK) level in the blood.
- Minor elevations of CK are common and may not relate to statin treatment.
- Severe myositis or rhabdomyolysis is rare.
- Myalgia can be reduced by lowering the dose of statin, adding in other treatment, or changing to another statin.

11.1 Biochemistry of CK

CK is an enzyme found widely throughout the body, wherever energy exchange is taking place. It facilitates the reversible reaction:

Phosphocreatine + ADP + proton ↔ creatine + ATP

CK is a dimeric protein, with two subunits named either M (muscle) or B (brain). In skeletal muscle, most of the CK is in the isoform MM, and the brain, BB. In the heart, up to 40% is the mixed form MB, unique to cardiac tissue. In the circulation, most of the total CK (tCK) measured is the MM isoform, with <5% MB and very little BB. Because the mass of skeletal muscle tissue is so great, tCK is a very sensitive measure of muscle damage.

Levels are very high in patients with inflammatory or metabolic muscle disease, and even modest exercise or trauma can produce a detectable increase. Other causes of an elevated tCK include CNS disease such as stroke or intracranial haemorrhage, cardiopulmonary disease such as myocardial infarction, bowel infarction, pulmonary embolism and pneumonia, and metabolic causes such as shock, sepsis, and hypothyroidism. In addition, tCK levels may be elevated due to the presence of a macroenzyme (Lee *et al.*, 1994), which usually migrates with the MB fraction on electrophoresis. This is thought to be a normal variant. There are therefore many potential causes for a raised tCK in the blood, and not all indicate a serious problem.

11.2 **Clinical features**

Most lipid-lowering drugs, including statins, fibrates, and nicotinic acid, have been described as causing muscle problems. At one end of the spectrum is myalgia, a subjective ache in the muscles without tenderness or other physical signs, and usually with a normal circulating tCK level, although this could be raised due to the causes noted earlier. Myositis is characterized by severe generalized muscle pains, accompanied by an elevation of tCK to at least five times the upper limit of normal. There is often muscle tenderness. It can progress to frank rhabdomyolysis with myoglobinuria, glomerular damage, and ultimately renal failure (Sathasivam and Lecky, 2008).

There do seem to be predisposing factors to the development of myositis (see Table 9.4). Hypothyroidism is an independent cause of a raised tCK (see above) and should be treated before any lipid-lowering medications are given—this alone can normalize the cholesterol levels. Renal impairment, and the use of immunosuppressant drugs such as ciclosporin, can also predispose to myositis.

The likelihood of developing muscle problems varies from one statin to another and to a certain extent depends on the metabolism of the drug (see Chapter 9; Law and Rudnicka, 2006). Cerivastatin was more prone than the others to cause problems, especially when combined with gemfibrozil (Bermingham et al., 2000), and has since been withdrawn (Furberg and Pitt, 2001; Psaty et al., 2004). There have also been concerns about the use of rosuvastatin (Alsheikh-Ali et al., 2005). With other drugs such as simvastatin, the risk of myositis appears to be dose-related (Waters, 2005). Overall, the incidence of myositis is low, and rhabdomyolysis occurs in <1 in 10,000 patients (Armitage, 2007). A genomewide scan has indicated that a single-nucleotide polymorphism (SNP) in the gene encoding for the soluble carrier organic anion transporter family, member 1B1 (*SLCO1B1*) may predispose to the development of myopathy (SEARCH, 2008) and so in the future it may be possible to screen patients before starting treatment.

Whilst true myositis may be rare, aches and pains are of course very common, and there are also many reasons why there should be small elevations of tCK in the blood (see above). To be confident about the diagnosis of myositis, then in addition to these widespread severe pains, there should a considerable elevation in circulating tCK, usually to >1000 IU/L. Either feature alone cannot sustain the diagnosis, and it is important to be confident before recommending withdrawal of treatment, as for many patients, lipid-lowering treatment is part of their therapeutic regime. *Whilst it is important to maintain vigilance for the adverse effects of drugs, it is also important not to blame drugs if they are innocent.*

11.3 **Use of ubiquinone**

Inhibition of HMG-CoA reductase by statins not only reduces the intracellular levels of mevalonate and cholesterol, especially in the liver, but also reduces the level of the ubiquinone coenzyme Q10 (CoQ10; Hargreaves, 2003). CoQ10 is an electron carrier in the mitochondrial respiratory chain, and an important intracellular antioxidant. It may protect LDL-C against oxidation (Berliner and Heinecke, 1996; Thomas *et al.*, 1999) and hence prevent the onset of atherosclerosis (see Chapter 5). Levels of CoQ10 are low in patients with coronary artery disease (Hanaki *et al.*, 1993) or hyperlipidaemia (Kontush *et al.*, 1997). Levels are reduced by statins but not fibrates, and an increased blood lactate/pyruvate ratio indicated possible mitochondrial dysfunction (De Pinieux *et al.*, 1996). There is therefore a theoretical background to the development of muscle problems after statin therapy (Nawarkas, 2005).

Reduced CoQ10 levels after pravastatin do not appear to be associated with an unfavourable outcome (Stocker *et al.*, 2006), and there is no clear evidence that restoring plasma levels of CoQ10 by supplementation is of benefit, especially in the relief of symptoms (Reidenberg, 2005; Marcoff and Thompson, 2007). Randomized controlled trials (RCTs) of coenzyme Q10 supplementation are few and small-scale (Caso *et al.*, 2007), and so most of the evidence is anecdotal.

11.4 **Clinical implications**

We would strongly recommend that a baseline tCK (as well as liver function tests including γ-glutamyltranspeptidase, GGT) be measured before initiating lipid-lowering therapy. If the levels of tCK are only modestly elevated, and there is an explanation (such as heavy exercise) then it is usually safe to proceed, monitoring the tCK levels every 3 months or so, or if there is a complaint of muscle pain. If the patient has a very high baseline tCK level, suggestive of underlying muscle disease, then specialist advice should be sought, although the possibility of treatment is not completely excluded. If the patient develops aches and pains whilst on treatment, it is important that such treatment is not withdrawn until a blood sample for tCK has been taken as it is difficult to establish innocence in retrospect.

References

Alsheikh-Ali AA, Ambrose MS, Kuvin JT, and Karas RH (2005). The safety of rosuvastatin as used in common clinical practice. A postmarketing analysis. *Circulation*, **111**, 3051–7.

Armitage J (2007). The safety of statins in clinical practice. *Lancet*, **370**, 1781–90.

Berliner JA and Heinecke JW (1996). The role of oxidized lipoproteins in atherogenesis. *Free Radic. Biol. Med.*, **20**, 707–27.

Bermingham RP, Whitsitt TB, Smart ML *et al.* (2000). Rhabdomyolysis in a patient receiving the combination of cerivastatin and gemfibrozil. *Am. J. Health-Syst. Pharm.*, **57**, 461–4.

Caso G, Kelly P, McNurlan M and Lawson W, (2007). Effect of coenzyme Q10 on myopathic symptoms in patients treated with statins. *Am. J. Cardiol.*, **99**: 1409–12.

De Pinieux G, Chariot P, Ammi-Saïd M *et al.* (1996). Lipid-lowering drugs and mitochondrial function: effects of HMG-CoA reductase inhibitors on serum ubiquinone and blood lactate/pyruvate ratio. *Br. J. Clin. Pharmacol.*, **42**, 333–7.

Furberg CD and Pitt B (2001). Withdrawal of cerivastatin from the world market. *Curr. Control. Trials Cardiovasc. Med.*, **2**, 205–7.

Hanaki Y, Sugiyama S, Ozawa T, and Ohno M (1993). Coenzyme Q_{10} and coronary artery disease. *Clin. Invest.*, **71**, S112–S115.

Hargreaves IP (2003). Ubiquinone—cholesterol's reclusive cousin. *Ann. Clin. Biochem.*, **40**, 207–18.

Kontush A, Reich A, Baum K *et al.* (1997). Plasma ubiquinol-1 is decreased in patients with hyperlipidaemia. *Atherosclerosis*, **128**, 119–26.

Law M and Rudnicka AR (2006). Statin safety: a systematic review. *Am. J. Cardiol.*, **97**, 52C–62C.

Lee KN, Csako G, Bernhardt P, and Elim RJ (1994). Relevance of macro creatine kinase type 1 and 2 isoenzymes to laboratory and clinical data. *Clin. Chem.*, **40**, 1278–83.

Marcoff L and T–hompson PD (2007). The role of coenzyme Q10 in statin-induced myopathy. *J. Am. Coll. Cardiol.*, **49**: 2231–7.

Nawarkas JJ (2005). HMG-CoA reductase inhibitors and coenzyme Q_{10}. *Cardiol. Rev.*, **13**, 76–9.

Psaty BM, Furberg CD, Ray WA *et al.* (2004). Potential for conflict of interest in the evaluation of suspected adverse drug reactions. Use of cerivastatin and risk of rhabdomyolysis. *J. Am. Med. Assoc.*, **292**, 2622–31.

Reidenberg MM (2005). Statins, lack of energy and ubiquinone. *Br. J. Clin. Pharmacol.*, **59**, 606–7.

Sathasivam S and Lecky B (2008). Statin induced myopathy. *Br. Med. J.*, **337**: 1159–62.

SEARCH Collaborative Group (2008). *SLCO1B1* variants and statin-induced myopathy—a genomewide study. *N. Engl. J. Med.*, **359**: 789–99.

Stocker R, Pollicino C, Gay CA *et al.* (2006). Neither plasma coenzyme Q_{10} concentration, not its decline during pravastatin therapy, is linked to recurrent cardiovascular disease events: a prospective case–control study from the LIPID study. *Atherosclerosis*, **187**, 198–204.

Thomas SR, Witting PK, and Stocker R (1999). The role of coenzyme Q in atherosclerosis. *Biofactors*, **9**, 207–24.

Waters DD (2005). Safety of high-dose atorvastatin therapy. *Am. J. Cardiol.*, **96**, 69F–75F.

Chapter 12

Lipid drug trials

Over the past 40 yrs there have been many studies into the clinical efficacy of lipid-lowering drugs, and assessment of their effects on morbidity and mortality both in patients with known coronary disease (*secondary prevention*) and in those without (*primary prevention*). The following does not attempt to be an exhaustive list, but is our personal choice of the most influential studies, that probably make up over 90% of our knowledge base in this area.

12.1 Non-statin studies

12.1.1 WHO (1978)

World Health Organisation: A co-operative trial in the primary prevention of ischaemic heart disease using clofibrate. Report(s) from the Committee of Principal Investigators (1978). Br. Heart J., 40, 1069–118; (1980). Lancet, ii, 379–85.

The first major international collaborative study suffered from teething problems. Cholesterol was reduced by 9% and non-fatal coronary events by 25% ($P < 0.05$), but there was an increase in all-cause mortality (also $P < 0.05$), mainly related to gastrointestinal malignancy. This cast a cloud over lipid treatment for many years, not fully dispelled until the 4S study (see below). It is now thought that the original data could be reworked and come to a different conclusion.

12.1.2 CDP (1975, 1986)

Coronary Drug Projects The CDP Research Group. (1975). J. Am. Med. Assoc., 231, 360–81. Canner PL et al. (1986). J. Am. Coll. Cardiol., 8, 1245–55.

The CDP groups were set up by the US Government in the 1950s to investigate the claims of various drugs to benefit heart disease. Early studies soon excluded D-thyroxine and oestrogen, and resins and nicotinic acid went on to more detailed analysis. The second study reports observations after 15 yrs of treatment with nicotinic acid and shows a mortality benefit in the active treatment group.

12.1.3 **LRC-CPPT (1984)**

Lipid Research Clinics Program Coronary Primary Prevention Trial.
LRC Program (1984). J. Am. Med. Assoc., 251, 351–64.

Despite the difficulties in placebo control, this trial showed reduced coronary events after treatment with the resin cholestyramine, but the statistical method used (one-tailed *t*-test) was inappropriate. No reduction in mortality was demonstrated.

12.1.4 **HHS (1987)**

Helsinki Heart Study. Frick MH et al. (1987). N. Engl. J. Med.,
317, 1237–45.

This study compared the effects of a fibrate (gemfibrozil) and placebo in a group of asymptomatic Finnish men with low-density lipoprotein cholesterol (LDL-C) >200 mg/dL (about 5 mmol/L). There was an impressive reduction in cardiovascular (CV) events (−34%) but again no reduction in mortality. The most benefit was seen in patients with insulin resistance syndromes and type 2 diabetes.

12.1.5 **VA-HIT (1999)**

Veteran's Affairs Cooperative Studies Program. Bloomfield RH et al.
(1999). N. Engl. J. Med., 341, 410–8.

This study describes the use of gemfibrozil in men with coronary disease and an high-density lipoprotein cholesterol (HDL-C) <1 mmol/L. A modest 23% event reduction was demonstrated, with no mortality benefit. Again, diabetics seemed to benefit most.

12.1.6 **BIP (2000)**

Bezafibrate Infarction Prevention study. BIP Study Group (2000).
Circulation, 102, 21–7.

Designed to address the relative lack of objective data on the beneficial effect of fibrates, this secondary prevention study showed an 18% increase in HDL-C levels and a reduction in high triglyceride (TG) levels, but no significant effect on CV morbidity or mortality. Many patients were lost to follow-up during the study.

12.1.7 **FIELD (2005)**

Fenofibrate Intervention and Event Lowering in Diabetes, FIELD
Study Investigators (2005). Lancet, 366, 1849–61.

A large-scale study of 9795 diabetic patients given fenofibrate or placebo, mean age 62 yrs and total cholesterol (TC) 3.0–6.5 mmol/L. Non-fatal myocardial infarction (MI) or death from coronary heart disease (CHD) occurred in 5.2% on active treatment and 5.9% on placebo (*P* = 0.16). Some reduction in retinal problems.

12.2 **Statins—secondary prevention**

12.2.1 **4S (1994)**

Scandinavian Simvastatin Survival Study (1994). Lancet, 344, 1383–9.
A landmark study in the lipid field. In a study of 4444 patients (men and women) with CHD, simvastatin 20 mg daily produced a 25% reduction in TC, a 35% reduction in LDL-C, and an 8% increase in HDL-C. Simvastatin reduced new major CV events by 34% (28% vs 19%, P <0.00001) and overall mortality by 30% (12% vs 8%, P <0.0003). Most of the benefit was due to LDL-C reduction, and some due to an increase in HDL-C. Furthermore, economic analysis showed the treatment to be cost effective. With the publication of this study, all doubts about the value of lipid lowering in patients with CHD were removed.

12.2.2 **CARE (1996)**

Cholesterol And Recurrent Events trial, Sacks FM et al. (1996).
N. Engl. J. Med., 335, 1001–9.
In 4159 patients with an MI <20 months previously and a TC of <240 mg/dL (about 6 mmol/L), pravastatin 40 mg daily reduced fatal and non-fatal new CV events by 24% compared to placebo (P <0.003). An apparent increase in cancer (breast) was not confirmed in later studies such as LIPID (*qv*).

12.2.3 **LIPID (1998)**

Long-term Intervention with Pravastatin in Ischemic Disease, LIPID Study Group (1998). N. Engl. J. Med., 339, 1349–57.
Patients (n = 9014) with acute MI or recent unstable angina, TC 4–7 mmol/L were given dietary advice and pravastatin 40 mg daily or placebo. Over 6 yrs, deaths from CHD (6.4% vs 8.3%, P <0.001) and overall mortality (11.0% vs 14.1%, P <0.001) were reduced in the active treatment group.

12.2.4 **HPS (2002)**

MRC/BHF Heart Protection Study of cholesterol lowering with simvastatin in 20 536 high-risk individuals: a randomised placebo-controlled trial. Heart Protection Study Collaborative Group (2002). Lancet, 360, 7–21.
Patients with coronary disease, other vascular disease or diabetes were given simvastatin 40 mg daily or placebo for 5 yrs. All-cause mortality was reduced from 14.7% to 12.9% in the active treatment group (P = 0.0003), and many CV end points were reduced too. This benefit extended to patients with TC <5 mmol/L on inclusion.

12.2.5 **PROSPER (2002)**

*Prospective study of Pravastatin in the Elderly at Risk (2002). Lancet, **360**, 1623–30.*

Patients (n = 5804, mean age 75 yrs) with pre-existing vascular disease or at risk due to smoking, hypertension, or diabetes, with TC 4–9 and TG <6 mmol/L were given dietary advice and pravastatin 40 mg daily or placebo. Over 3.2 yrs, new CV events occurred in 14.1% on active treatment and 16.2% on placebo (P = 0.014). The benefit was mainly in heart diseases. There was no improvement in stroke rate, and cognition did not benefit. Any change in cognition related to apo E isoform rather than TC levels.

12.3 **Statins—primary prevention**

12.3.1 **WOSCOPS (1995)**

*West of Scotland Coronary Prevention Study, Shepherd J et al. (1995). N. Engl. J. Med., **333**, 1301–7.*

Asymtomatic men (n = 6595) aged 45–64 yrs were followed up for nearly 5 yrs. Their initial TC was <6 and LDL-C <4 mmol/L, and they were given pravastatin 40 mg daily or placebo. Clearly some of the men had silent coronary disease, and this may have contributed to the significant reductions in new CV events, fatal and non-fatal MI. The 22% reduction in all-cause mortality just failed to reach significance (P = 0.051). This is an important study because of its large-scale and careful monitoring. A subsequent 12-yr follow-up showed continuing benefit in the active treatment group, even though treatment had not been continued.

12.3.2 **AFCAPS/TexCAPS (1998)**

*Air Force/Texas Coronary Atherosclerosis Prevention Study, Downs JR et al. (1998). J. Am. Med. Assoc., **279**, 1615–22.*

Another large-scale study involving 6605 men and women, followed up for nearly 5 yrs and treated diet and with lovastatin (20 or 40 mg daily, according to LDL-C levels) or placebo. Their mean baseline TC was 5.7 mmol/L and HDL-C 0.94 in men and 1.03 mmol/L in women. Low HDL-C was the main driver to recruitment. TC levels were reduced by 18% on treatment, and HDL-C increased by 6%. New CV events were reduced by 37% (P <0.001) and so were several other CV end points, but not overall mortality.

12.3.3 **ASCOT-LLA (2003)**

*Anglo-Scandinavian Cardiac Outcomes Trial—Lipid Lowering Arm, Sever PS et al. (2003). Lancet, **361**, 1149–58.*

A large study comparing anti-hypertensive medications in one arm, and the benefits of added lipid-lowering medication in another. In the second arm, 10,305 patients with treated hypertension, TC <6.5 mmol/L were given atorvastatin 10 mg daily or placebo and followed for up to 5 yrs. Fatal or non-fatal CHD occurred on 1.9% of the statin group and 3.0% on placebo ($P = 0.0005$), and the study was discontinued. The risk profile of the patients in this study was similar to WOSCOPS (*qv*).

12.3.4 **CARDS (2004)**

Collaborative Atorvastatin Diabetes Study, Colhoun HM et al. (2004). Lancet, **364***, 685–96.*

Patients (*n* = 2838) with type 2 diabetes, LDL-C <4.0 mmol/L, TG <6.8 mmol/L and one other risk factor for CHD were given atorvastatin 10 mg daily or placebo in addition to their usual treatment. Over nearly 4 yrs, new CV events occurred in 5.8% on statin and 9.0% on placebo ($P = 0.001$), a relative risk reduction of 37%.

12.3.5 **JUPITER (2008)**

Rosuvastatin to prevent vascular events in men and women with elevated C-reactive protein. Ridker PM, et al. (2008) N. Engl. J. Med., **359***: 2195–2207.*

In 17,802 subjects with no history of vascular disease and normal lipid levels, those with a high-sensitivity CRP (hsCRP) level of >2 mg/l (a surrogate marker for inflammation in the arteries) were randomly assigned to rosuvastatin 20 mg daily or placebo. After a mean follow-up time of <2 years, when the trial was discontinued on the advice of the Ethics Review Board, active treatment had reduced LDL-C levels by 50%, hsCRP by 37%, vascular events (hazard ratio 0.53; 95% CI 0.40–0.69; P <0.00001) and all-cause mortality. The clinical (and financial) implications of this large-scale study have yet to be decided.

12.4 **High vs low dose statin**

12.4.1 **STELLAR (2003)**

Comparison of the efficacy and safety of rosuvastatin versus atorvastatin, simvastatin, and pravastatin across doses. Jones PH et al. (2003) Am. J. Cardiol., **93***, 152–60.*

Head-to-head comparison of the recommended doses of four statins in 2431 patients with LDL-C in the range 160–250 mg/dL. The order of potency was rosuvastatin >atorvastatin >simvastatin >pravastatin. LDL-C was reduced to <3 mmol/L in 79%–92% on rosuvastatin. Tolerability was similar for the four drugs. Note that was a short-term (6 week) efficacy study and there are no data on long-term effects.

12.4.2 **PROVE IT–TIMI 22 (2004)**

Pravastatin or atorvastatin Evaluation and Infection Therapy Thrombolysis in Myocardial Infarction, Cannon CP et al. (2004). N. Engl. J. Med., 350, 1495–504.

C-reactive protein levels and outcomes after statin therapy, Ridker PM et al. (2005). N. Engl. J. Med., 352, 20–8.

Patients with acute MI or ACS (*n* = 4162), mean age 58 yrs and TC <6.2 mmol/L, were given pravastatin 40 mg or atorvastatin 80 mg daily, with a possible dose increment of pravastatin to 80 mg if LDL-C was still >3 mmol/L. They were also given antibiotic (gatifloxacin) or placebo. New CV events were recorded in 26.3% on pravastatin and 22.4% on atorvastatin (*P* = 0.005). Greater reductions in LDL-C were associated with greater benefit. There was no difference between the active antibiotic and placebo groups, but C-reactive protein (CRP) was a strong predictor of outcome.

12.4.3 **A to Z (2004)**

Aggrastat to Zocor. de Lemos JA et al. (2004). J. Am. Med. Assoc., 292, 1307–16.

The first part of this study compared enoxaparin and unfractionated heparin in the treatment of NSTEMI/ACS. The second part (Phase Z) compared the effect in 4497 such patients of initiating simvastatin 40 mg daily early, increasing after a month to 80 mg, with a placebo for 4 months followed by 20 mg daily. After 2 yrs, there was no significant difference in new CV events between the two groups. This is a complicated study, difficult to analyse.

12.4.4 **TNT (2004)**

Treating to New Targets, Waters DD et al. (2004). Am. J. Cardiol., 93, 154–8; (2005). N. Engl. J. Med., 352, 1425–35.

Wenger NK et al. (2008). Heart, 94, 434–9.

In patients with stable CHD and LDL-C <3.4 mmol/L (*n* = 10 001), levels were reduced to 2.6 mmol/L by atorvastatin 10 mg and to 2.0 mmol/L by 80 mg. After nearly 5 yrs, the composite CV end point occurred in 10.9% on low dose and 8.7% on high dose (relative risk reduction 22%, *P* <0.001). There was no difference in overall mortality, but the study was not powered to demonstrate this. A later report has confirmed similar findings in women.

12.4.5 **IDEAL (2005)**

Incremental Decrease in Endpoints through Aggressive Lipid lowering (2005). J. Am. Med. Assoc., 294, 2437–45.

Patients with a history of MI (*n* = 8888) were given atorvastatin 80 or simvastatin 20–40 mg daily. The difference in the composite CV end point just failed to reach significance between the two groups

(P = 0.07) but the trends are similar to the outcomes from TNT (see above).

12.4.6 REVERSAL (2005)

*Nissen SE et al. (2005). Statin therapy, LDL cholesterol, C-reactive protein, and coronary artery disease. N. Engl. J. Med., **352**, 29–38.*

Coronary intravascular ultrasound (IVUS) was carried out in 502 patients before and after 18 months of moderate lipid-lowering treatment (pravastatin 40 mg daily) or more intensive treatment (atorvastatin 80 mg). The reduced rate of progression observed after intensive treatment related both to greater reduction of LDL-C and to CRP levels.

Chapter 13

Clinical cases

These are 20 recent real cases from the Lipid Clinic and represent many of the common problems encountered.

1. **A lady aged 46 is found to have TC of 6.5 mmol/L at a works screening programme. She has no other risk factors for cardiovascular disease.**
   She is at low risk for a cardiovascular (CV) event over the next 10 yrs and so she should be offered lifestyle advice rather than active treatment.

2. **A man aged 56 is found to have TC of 6.5 mmol/L, HDL-C 1.1 mmol/L, as part of a Well Man clinic. He smokes 20 cigarettes a day and his blood pressure is 160/90 mmHg.**
   The probability of a CV event over the next 10 yrs is >20%, and so if the lipid profile is confirmed he should be started on generic simvastatin 20 mg daily, increasing to 40 mg if needed. The initial target is a total cholesterol (TC) of <5 mmol/L and an LDL-C of <3 mmol/L. Ideally his cholesterol levels should be <4 and <2, respectively.

3. **A man aged 65 has recently developed angina, and during angiography had PTCA to two vessels, and stents were deployed. He is normotensive and does not smoke.**
   He has TC 5.6 mmol/L, LDL-C 3.4 mmol/L, and HDL-C 1.6 mmol/L. In the presence of known coronary disease, the cholesterol should be aggressively treated to the lower targets above.

4. **A man aged 54 had CABG 3 yrs ago and his cholesterol is 6.5 mmol/L on simvastatin 40 mg daily.**
   This level of control is unacceptable. Possible treatment strategies include to change to a more potent statin such as atorvastatin or rosuvastatin, or add ezetimibe, or both.

5. **A lady aged 26 presents with a cholesterol of 12.5 mmol/L. Her father died suddenly at 32 and she thinks her brother has 'a cholesterol problem'.**
   This is almost certainly familial hypercholesterolaemia (FH). The diagnosis would be confirmed by the presence of tendon xanthomata in the patients or a close relative, but often this evidence is lacking. Nevertheless a full family screen is indicated, and genetic testing if available. The patient should be on active

treatment to the targets above. Simvastatin is unlikely to reach these targets and so start with atorvastatin or rosuvastatin. Contraceptive advice should be offered, and treatment withheld if pregnancy is actively sought.

6. **A boy of 10 has genetically proven FH and there is a bad family history of premature vascular disease. His cholesterol is 7.5 mmol/L.**
   There is convincing evidence of vascular disease in children with FH, even by the age of 11 with pravastatin or atorvastatin. He should be on active treatment.

7. **A lady aged 53 is on simvastatin 20 mg following the discovery of a cholesterol of 6.1 mmol/L and no other risk factors for CV disease. She complains of generalized aches and pains, and there are no objective signs of arthritis.**
   Measure the CK. Myositis is the only major adverse effect of statins, but is highly unlikely if the CK level is normal. Sometimes changing to another statin helps, but in this case there is a question over whether treatment is needed at all.

8. **A man aged 55 is on atorvastatin 40 mg following CABG 10 yrs previously. His TC is 5.8 mmol/L, with an LDL-C of 3.9 mmol/L. He complains of aches and pains and his CK is 232 IU/L (normal <150).**
   Minor elevations in CK are common, and may occur after injury or unaccustomed exertion. In addition, a minority of patients have a high CK to start with, often due to the presence of a macroenzyme. Clearly there is an imperative to active treatment here and so every effort should be made to find a treatment combination that reaches targets but does not cause discomfort.

9. **A lady aged 25 with FH is being treated with atorvastatin 40 mg daily. On routine testing her CK is 4500 IU/L but she has no muscle pains.**
   Her CK before treatment was known to be normal. Very high levels can occur after unusual exercise. In this case, she had taken part in a half-Marathon 3 days previously.

10. **A man aged 53 has a cholesterol of 8.2 mmol/L and a CK of 3400 IU/L before treatment. He admits to fatigue and leg pains on exertion and so does not perform any strenuous exercise.**
    He was found to have the rare metabolic muscle disease McArdle's Syndrome (myophosphorylase deficiency). Such patients may develop premature CV disease and so he probably should be treated, but under close supervision.

11. **A lady of 46 develops an AST of 83 and an ALT of 95 IU/L after starting on rosuvastatin 10 mg. The pre-treatment levels were normal, and she is asymptomatic.**

Minor elevations of liver enzymes are common on statin treatment, and should not cause concern unless they exceed three times the upper limit of normal. From extended post-marketing surveillance over a 20-yr period we know that statin therapy is not associated with liver disease or failure.

12. **After starting simvastatin 20 mg in a lady of 53, her GGT level increased from 54 to 432 IU/L.**

There is no relationship of statins to γGT and so another cause should be sought. Measure her viral and general antibody status and request an ultrasound scan of the upper abdomen.

13. **A man of 46 presents with a cholesterol of 7.5 mmol/L and a fasting triglyceride (TG) of 4.6 mmol/L.**

This lipid profile is frequently observed secondary to other causes, such as diabetes, obesity, excess alcohol intake, and thyroid or renal disease. These should be excluded before treatment, which is best with a fibrate rather than a statin.

14. **A lady aged 20 is found to have lipaemic plasma, and her fasting TG was 56 mmol/L.**

Such patients are at great risk of potentially fatal pancreatitis. She should be admitted for a low fat diet, fibrates, and marine oils until levels have fallen to <10 mmol/L. Other members of the family should be screened for the same condition, which may relate to lipoprotein lipase deficiency. Haemofiltration may be needed. Particular problems may occur during pregnancy, when the lipid profile tends to be worse.

15. **A man aged 54 has a total cholesterol of 5.3 mmol/L, an HDL-C of 0.75 mmol/L, and a fasting TG of 4.5 mmol/L. He does not smoke and his blood pressure and blood glucose are normal.**

This combination is a potentially atherogenic lipid profile, and may occur secondary to diabetes. It should be treated with a fibrate or nicotinic acid.

16. **After starting the patient on fenofibrate 200 mg, his HDL-C level fell to 0.2 mmol/L.**

A steep fall in HDL-C occurs occasionally after fibrate treatment, and the mechanism is as yet unknown. Stop the fibrate and try nicotinic acid instead.

17. **Commencing nicotinic acid he complained of intolerable flushing and itching.**
    Flushing is a very common reaction to nicotinic acid tablets, but the problem is greatly reduced if treatment is introduced slowly, is taken before bedtime, and is preceded by aspirin, as the flush is prostacyclin-mediated. Tolerance develops over time, without loss of efficacy.

18. **A man aged 43 has a cholesterol of 8.4 mmol/L and a TG of 5.6 mmol/L. He describes yellow streaks on the palms of his hands. He is overweight at 96 kg, and after losing 5 kg on a diet, his lipid profile normalizes.**
    This sounds very much like remnant (type III) hyperlipidaemia, which can be very weight-sensitive. Confirm by finding his apo E genotype or phenotype to be E_2/E_2. Untreated it may lead to peripheral vascular disease, and the treatment of choice is a fibrate.

19. **A lady aged 64 has angina, and her blood pressure is 155/90 on treatment. She smokes 10 cigarettes a day. Her cholesterol is 7.5 mmol/L and she has tried many different treatments but none of them agree with her.**
    The first step is to agree with her that some form of treatment is needed, and to explain that there are now a wide range of options, so it is unusual to fail to find a combination that does not suit. The second step is to find the exact nature of her symptoms, and their temporal relationship to treatment, if any. Objective evidence, such as a normal CK in the presence of muscle aches, may help to reassure her. Unfortunately though there does remain a small minority of patients in whom no treatment appears to be tolerated and one can only focus on lifestyle advice, such as her stopping smoking.

20. **A man of 64 has maturity onset (type 2) diabetes and is on treatment with metformin 500 mg b.d. His glycaemic control is poor, with a fasting glucose of 12.5 mmol/L and HbA1c of 11%. His lipid profile is recorded as TC 6.3 mmol/L, HDL-C 0.8 mmol/L, and TG 3.4 mmol/L.**
    The sustained hyperglycaemia is making a major contribution to his abnormal lipids, and so this should be the first line of intervention. In the meantime, treatment is indicated, usually with a fibrate, or (if TC and LDL-C alone are elevated) a statin, to the targets noted above.

Useful links

British Cardiovascular Society
The new name for the British Cardiac Society reflects their wider interest
9 Fitzroy Square
London W1T 5HW
enquiries@bcs.com

British Heart Foundation
A major supporter of research in the cardiovascular area
14 Fitzhardinge Street
London W1H 6DH
www.bhf.org.uk

Heart UK
The amalgamation of the British Hyperlipidaemia Association and the patient-centred Family Heart Association, they have a special interest in familial hypercholesterolaemia (FH)
7 North Road
Maidenhead
Berks SL6 1PE
ask@heartuk.org.uk

Irish Cardiac Society
Includes the Irish Heart Foundation
4 Clyde Road
Dublin 4
slawlor@irishheart.ie

Northern Ireland Chest, Heart and Stroke
A local charity with a broad base but an interest in lipid problems
21 Dublin Road
Belfast BT2 7HB
mail@nichsa.com

Royal Society of Medicine

Specialist Lipid Forum has regular meetings to a high standard
1 Wimpole Street
London W1G 0AE
membership@rsm.ac.uk

Simon Broome Trust

Specializes in the study of FH. Contact Professor Andrew Neil at:
andrew.neil@dphpc.ox.ac.uk

Index